The FitMama™ Method

The Complete Guide to Confidence and Fitness for Birth

MARIE BEHENNA

SOUVENIR PRESS

NOTE TO READERS

This publication contains the ideas and opinions of its author. It is intended to provide helpful and informative material on the subjects addressed in the publication. It is sold with the understanding that the author and publisher are not engaged in rendering medical, health or any other kind of personal professional services in the book.

The reader should consult his or her medical, health or other competent professional before adopting any of the suggestions in this book or drawing inferences from it.

The author and publisher specifically disclaim all responsibility for any liability, loss or risk, personal or otherwise, which is incurred as a consequence, directly or indirectly, of the use and application of any of the contents of this book.

DEDICATION

For every woman who wants to feel empowered by knowledge, and for my children who have waited countless hours for me to finish 'just one more page'.

ISBN 9780285640863

Typeset by M Rules
Printed and bound by Bell & Bain Ltd., Glasgow

CONTENTS

SECTION ONE: WHAT, WHY AND WHO SAYS?

SECTION TWO: THE EXERCISE TECHNIQUES

FOREWORD

Miss Bronwyn Middleton Bell
MRCOG, MBChB, DFFP
Consultant Obstetrician and Gynaecologist
The Poundbury Clinic
Author of RCOG Statement 4: Exercise in Pregnancy
Gynaecologist for London Olympics 2012

I truly believe that empowering women with the tools to support them through pregnancy and labour reaps huge benefits in the outcomes achieved. This book is one of those tools.

Pregnancy should be recognised as a unique time for behaviour modification and is no longer considered a condition for confinement. It is clear that exercise in pregnancy and the post-natal period is beneficial to mum and baby with the right guidance. Pregnancy exercise should be a combination of aerobic, strength and resistance training, and muscular release. This combination will prepare your body for pregnancy itself as well as labour and the post-partum period. Marie Behenna has written *The FitMama™ Method* optimising the balance between nutrition, reducing stress levels and exercise. Marie even includes comprehensive advice to our partners on how to support us in labour.

We know that exercise has real benefit in preventing disease such as diabetes and heart disease. Many common complaints of pregnancy, including fatigue, varicosities and swelling of extremities, are reduced in women who exercise. Additionally, active women experience less insomnia, stress, anxiety and depression. There is some evidence that weight-bearing exercise throughout pregnancy can reduce the length of labour and decrease delivery complications. Women who incorporate exercise into their routine during pregnancy are more likely to continue exercising postpartum. Evidence also suggests a protective effect of exercise on heart disease, osteoporosis and high blood pressure as well as a reduced risk of colon cancer and breast cancer. There are certain circumstances when exercise is not indicated in pregnancy or when extra precautions should be taken and Marie provides clear guidance on these.

Marie is an inspiration to pregnant and postnatal women and their carers. Not only has she dedicated her life to learning about and promoting healthy pregnancies through nutrition and exercise, she has had the initiative to capture her insight in this book to share it with you.

I had the pleasure of meeting Marie, although slightly later than I would have chosen, when I was 6 weeks postnatal and raring to get back into some sort of physical exercise. I managed to remain 'low risk' throughout my pregnancy, despite my glaringly obvious risk factor of being a consultant obstetrician and gynaecologist. My water birth was an amazing experience and achievement next to no other.

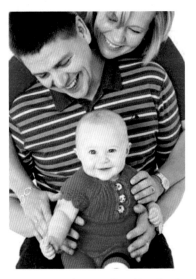

Not only did Marie's Postnatal Pelvic Floor Repair class encourage me to get back safely into pre-pregnancy shape, it also provided me with social interaction with women in similar circumstances. We didn't have to part with our newborns, they were safely by our side. Some classes were more challenging than others and that was just ensuring baby compliance and co-operation. We were all tired with new babies who craved our company 24/7, struggling to get it together to look half presentable to make it out the house, let alone exercise. We all wanted to be FitMamas. Sharing this was invaluable; benefits were immense and not only physical.

Bronwyn Middleton Bell and her family

This comprehensive book will empower you with invaluable knowledge to confidently enjoy the benefits of staying fit and healthy in preparation for motherhood and beyond. The rewards of following this advice will be enormous, both physically and psychologically.

Healthy, happy FitMama = healthy, happy FitBaba and family . . . we deserve it!

INTRODUCTION

When people ask me what I do, I am used to receiving quizzical looks when I tell them that I coach women in pregnancy exercise and techniques for delivery. Those who have no experience of coming across pregnant women look at me as though I am joking. Some think I am extremely brave for having these creatures within two feet of me when they could explode into labour at any moment! But those women who have experienced pregnancy will be very interested; many will say how they wish my services had been around when they were pregnant.

I feel thoroughly blessed to have found this path in life, and am yet to have one of my ladies begin labour during any of my sessions. (Although I secretly carry an emergency delivery pack with me, just in case. Always be prepared!)

To prepare you for birth, this book will not only cover exercises, healing recipes and meditations for pregnancy, but will also teach you breathing and labour techniques to help you feel in control during the birth itself. Some of our wonderful former FitMama™ participants also share their stories with you in this book – amusing, informative and extremely grounding.

There is a lot of debate about whether to exercise before twelve weeks gestation, but I believe pregnancy is a natural state of being and that therefore exercise is good for you and your developing baby. Exercise will help your circulation flow more easily, taking nutrients to your baby and keeping your organs well looked after. I encourage women at *all* stages of pregnancy to exercise. As long as you are listening to your body, you will always know when it is time to rest. Historically, women have worked the fields and rice paddies for thousands of years in all stages of pregnancy, sometimes giving birth in the field. We need to unite as women and mothers and embrace exercise positively. We are the field workers of the modern world.

The exercise methods in this book are designed simply to keep you mobile and active, and help you avoid too much strain on the body as your pregnancy progresses. This simple programme is appropriate at any stage of pregnancy, at any fitness level, and is designed to make you feel better. If you find anything gives you pain or makes you feel unwell, you must stop and seek advice from your midwife.

You will notice that our beautiful model Lola (also a FitMama™ trainer) is very heavily pregnant in the photographs throughout this book. But *The FitMama™ Method* is written with all of you in mind, at every stage of pregnancy. So even if your bump is nowhere near showing as much as Lola's yet, these exercises are still for you.

I have written this book with one main goal in mind: to give you confidence and self-awareness, so that when you enter your labour you will feel comfortable in your own pregnant skin. I want you to feel confident that your body will do what it needs to do to get your baby out of your womb and into your loving arms.

From one mother to another: listen to the advice given to you; apply it *only* if it works for you; take every dramatic birth story with a pinch of salt (no point in frightening yourself with what if's); and remember that every labour and birth experience is different.

You're already doing the right thing by learning more about yourself by picking up this book!

All my best wishes to you for a smooth and active pregnancy.

Marie Behenna

What, why and who says?

CHAPTER 1

It started with a kiss

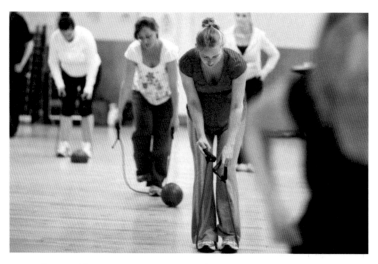

FitMama™ participants, November 2010, courtesy Carli-Art.co.uk

Ever since I was a young girl, I have been intrigued by pregnant women. I used to pass a pregnancy exercise studio on my walk home from school, and I would press my nose against the window to get a glimpse of these amazing women. I wanted to be like them one day, going through the motions of keeping well during this spectacular, life-creating period of their lives. I was completely unaware how this fascination would evolve into a passion for me once motherhood came into my own life.

My own journey began on a sunny winter's day in London Docklands, as I sat in great anticipation for my first home visit from my new midwife. (Yes, in those days we had home visits!) I was brimming with excitement, anxious to hear what she had to say and what wonderful advice she would share with me. When the doorbell rang, I leaped from the sofa and rushed to the door to let her in. A lovely lady, with an aura of wise woman about her, strolled into my lounge and sat down with her folder on her lap. I bounded in behind her with my 13-week-old bump on board, only to be stopped in my tracks with her unexpected words: 'Sit down, my dear!' Stunned, I sat beside her on the sofa, at which point she poked me on the shoulder and said, 'Now sit back and put your feet up! You must not exert yourself!'

In those days, I was a young and naïve city worker. I did as I was told, finding it difficult to relax to the extent she had indicated. But eventually, pregnancy tiredness took over and I gave in. However, my natural desire to exercise came storming back the day I went into labour with my baby boy, and I was overcome with a desire to break into a sprint while walking my dogs. Hey presto! The start of labour!

But that one moment of exercise was not enough to prepare me for the exertion of delivery. After 26 hours, and threats of forceps, I finally managed to push my 7lb 3oz baby out, with severe tearing. Ouch! No one tells you how hard the pushing is – but that is another conversation for later in this book.

Seven years later, my experience delivering my 8lb 13oz baby girl was the complete opposite. Fortunately, opinions within the midwifery and gynaecological fields had evolved since my first pregnancy, and I was not encouraged to simply put my feet up, relax and eat for two. On the contrary, I was encouraged to exercise throughout my pregnancy. I walked twice a day, every day, up and down a steep hill to take my son to and from school, then rested while he was at school (I had lost my job in early pregnancy, so had the luxury of rest time). I took much more notice of my pelvic floor muscles, and paid attention to my food consumption – although my cravings for chocolate and gold top Jersey milk were overwhelming! My labour was more manageable, lasting only two hours; my recovery was so much quicker; and my milk flowed more freely than first time around.

Eleven months later, I embarked on my journey to bring knowledge and fitness to pregnant women everywhere. After qualifying to work with pregnant women in exercise classes, I spent all my free time researching pregnancy exercise, mobility and birthing techniques. I continue to attend regular workshops hosted by professionals in the field of maternity health and exercise.

After all my investigations, it is clear to me that exercise alone is not enough to give women the toolbox to a successful pregnancy, labour and delivery. Women need confidence and knowledge to understand how their labour and delivery will be affected by their health and wellbeing. Understanding simple facts, such as which muscles help to push a baby out, can give a labouring woman a great advantage as she uses her body to bring her child into this world.

As a pregnancy exercise and education specialist, I have worked with hundreds of pregnant women, helping them through their pregnancies and into motherhood. I witness the miracle of developing life on a daily basis. My life with these women was not an accident! It was born of a desire to give women what I wanted during *my* pregnancies: knowledge, choice, confidence and fitness for childbirth.

LESSONS TO SHARE

- Keeping fit and healthy makes all the difference to the comfort and confidence of labour and delivery.
- Understanding your body will help to get your baby out.
- Breathing correctly is the accelerator for pushing.
- There is no set formula for a perfect delivery.
- Your body knows what to do, your baby knows how to be born: use the tools you have to give body and baby a smoother ride.
- Share this knowledge with other mums to prevent unnecessary complications during pregnancy and delivery and to empower women everywhere!

STAND UP AND TAKE NOTICE

So what is the evidence behind exercising during pregnancy? Research has proven that exercise during pregnancy is not only safe, but beneficial to the health and wellbeing of both mum and baby.

Helping to reduce the risk of gestational diabetes and high blood pressure, fitness during pregnancy also gives mums the physical advantage in actual delivery. A fitter mum finds she can push her baby out with more confidence and less strain on the heart. A healthy heart can handle the intensity of pushing far more easily than a heart which has not been exercised and challenged during pregnancy.

WHAT IS GESTATIONAL DIABETES?

Gestational diabetes is diabetes that develops for the first time during pregnancy. It affects up to 14 per cent of mums-to-be.

Diabetes happens when your body can't produce enough of a hormone called insulin. Insulin is made by your pancreas, and it does two jobs: it regulates the amount of sugar available in your blood for energy, and it enables any sugar that isn't needed to be stored. During pregnancy, your body has to produce extra insulin to meet your baby's needs, especially from mid-pregnancy onwards. If your body can't manage this, you will have too much sugar in your blood. It's then that you may develop gestational diabetes.

Gestational diabetes usually goes away after your baby is born. It's unlike other types of diabetes, which are lifelong conditions. However, Type II diabetes is an increased risk if you have suffered from gestational diabetes.

A stronger mum can handle the ever-evolving pregnant shape, which, without strength and stability through exercise, can become a painful and restrictive burden. Mums who have continued to exercise their core abdominal muscles appropriately will find pushing far more effective. Based on feedback from my participants and the midwives I work with, I can say that mums with good levels of strength, stability and fitness will push for less time than mums who have not been active during pregnancy. It is impossible to convey to first-time mums how intense and difficult the pushing is. Pushing your baby out is probably one of the hardest natural challenges you will face in your healthy female physical life. I can only compare it to pushing a piano up a staircase by yourself, or running the London Marathon – and you would not contemplate running the London Marathon without training your body to complete the challenge. The same applies to pregnancy and delivery: train your body to cope with the challenge, and empower your pregnant mind with knowledge, understanding and self-awareness.

BEYOND YOUR CONTROL

There will always be women who have worked hard at staying healthy and well, but still require assistance during delivery – by forceps, ventouse, or emergency caesarean section. Sometimes events can be out of our control: for example, if your baby has broad shoulders and is facing the wrong way during delivery, this could require medical intervention, particularly if your baby becomes distressed. My method does not prevent you from needing assistance, but gives you the physical tools to better cope with any challenges your delivery poses. Imagine if you had not exercised or educated yourself at all: you would probably need assistance much sooner than if you had kept yourself aware, fit and strong.

What if you are planning a caesarean section anyway; does this mean you won't need to exercise or learn the breathing techniques? No: they will still be of benefit to you, because they'll aid your recovery from the surgical procedure. The breathing will help you to cope if you have stress in your pregnancy, and while having the anaesthetic administered for your caesarean section. These skills are completely transferable to your situation.

Knowledge is power, and is the key to facing delivery with calm confidence. This book is designed to help you find that natural womanly ability which is deep inside you. Women have been delivering babies since humans first evolved, and even though childbirth is now a clinical procedure you can still use your natural body and maternal instincts to help you survive the plethora of opinion and 'helpful' advice you will hear throughout your pregnancy and beyond. Use exercise to enjoy and empower the journey of your pregnancy and delivery!

Even if you fall into the category of women who cannot exercise during pregnancy, this book will show you some basic techniques to help you manage your labour more effectively.

UNDERSTANDING YOUR BODY

Aside from keeping fit and well during pregnancy, it is also essential to understand your body and how it works during labour. *The FitMama™ Method* will give you simple and straightforward explanations as to how your body works, what it needs and how to use it to your advantage. That includes muscles for pushing; breathing for pregnancy, labour and delivery; and relaxation techniques to help you and your baby find calm in what can be a very stressful time in your life.

Exercise and knowledge also help women to feel positive about the changes their body is undergoing. The natural endorphins released during exercise are good for both you and your baby. It is particularly hard to feel positive during the early stages when you feel ill and don't quite look pregnant, but all your clothes are too tight and it is perhaps too soon to tell the world. It's easy to feel down during this phase. Exercise will go some way to helping you focus on your growing baby and help you to feel better about yourself.

If you are exercising by attending a pregnancy excercise class, or with a group of pregnant friends and a trainer, you will find that the sense of community will help you get through the difficult times of your pregnancy too. It's not all about the physical changes; sometimes the support of other women going through the same as you is an incredible stabiliser during what can be an extremely emotional time. In the FitMama™ classes and groups women have forged long-term and meaningful friendships, and this gives me enormous fulfilment to observe – particularly in this modern world where families often live far away from each other, and the traditional support network of grandparents, aunties, sisters, your own mum, may not be close enough to help you through this time.

WHAT DO THE PROFESSIONAL BODIES SAY?

In support of guidelines from the American College of Obstetricians and Gynecologists, the Royal College of Obstetricians and Gynaecologists (RCOG) suggests that:

- All women should be encouraged to participate in aerobic and strength-conditioning exercise as part of a healthy lifestyle during their pregnancy.
- Reasonable goals of aerobic conditioning in pregnancy should be to maintain a good fitness level throughout pregnancy *without* trying to reach peak fitness level or train for athletic competition.
- Women should choose activities that will minimise the risk of loss of balance and foetal trauma (*no impact or contact sports*).
- Women should be advised that adverse pregnancy or neonatal outcomes are *not* increased for exercising women.
- Initiation of pelvic floor exercises in the immediate postpartum period may reduce the risk of future urinary incontinence.
- Women should be advised that moderate exercise during lactation *does not* affect the quantity or composition of breast milk or impact on foetal growth.

RCOG Online

Even though, during pregnancy, we will be faced with aches, pains, nausea, vomiting, cravings, emotional ups and downs, fears, anxiety, swelling, skin problems, vaginal discharge, gas and bloating, bleeding gums, constipation, excessive salivation, haemorrhoids, itchy skin, nosebleeds and yeast infections . . . it's still an amazing journey!

So, let's work together to take you forward into motherhood with calm confidence, and to use your empowered self to bring your child into this world.

The Royal College of Obstetricians and Gynaecologists publish information from their own research and from research undertaken by their peers in America. If you wish to see more scientific facts about exercise during pregnancy, you can view comprehensive reading materials from both organisations via the website www.rcog.org.uk

CHAPTER 2

So you think you can put your feet up and eat for two?

You may feel pressure, as many pregnant women do, to cancel your gym membership, eat for two, and fall prey to your cravings. Okay, some cravings are all right, but craving chocolate and apple pie is just asking for trouble!

Well-intended words of advice to eat up and take it easy are old wives' tales and myths that can cause us to put ourselves in a vulnerable position for delivery.

It is important to keep mobile and eat a wide variety of nutritious foods during pregnancy, and to take supplements if recommended by your health carer. Prenatal supplements will contain the appropriate levels of vitamins and minerals which help your body to curb your cravings. For example, if you crave chocolate, I have found that this is often an indication of low levels of magnesium in the system, among other nutrients.

I want you to avoid obesity during your pregnancy, and if you have entered pregnancy overweight already, then use the tips in this book to help avoid worsening your condition. Obesity in pregnancy will create extra work for your body, and make your pregnancy, labour and delivery so much more complicated. This book will help you find basic coping strategies and alternative options.

DID YOU KNOW?

Nutrition and diet have a lot to do with the development of stretch marks. A diet rich in zinc, vitamins A, D and C and protein can safeguard the quality of your skin as it adapts to your quickly-changing pregnant body. Hydration is also key in preventing stretch marks.

Below, you can see the official nutrition diagram as published by the Food Standards Agency in the UK. This is a clear guide to the kind of food balance you should be working into your maternal eating plan. It is never a good idea to go on extreme diets during pregnancy. Rather, find a good balance of healthy foods.

The Balance of Good Health

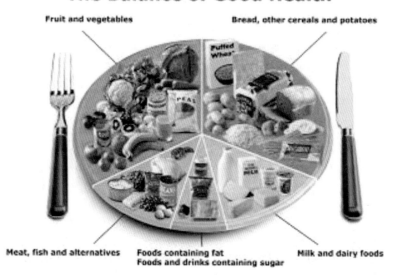

The balance of good health www.food.gov.uk

The 'balance of good health' template above is published by the Food Council as a guide to healthy eating. Some nutritionists, however, believe that the foods depicted on the plate aren't very good examples (for instance, white bread/pasta/rice are shown, whereas the wholemeal/wheat varieties would be better). The diagram is a good visual aid, but try to have less white starch, and more wholemeal and whole wheat as replacements.

If you are gluten, dairy, nut or egg intolerant, please seek advice from your health carer for suitable alternatives to the 'balance of good health' chart.

It is essential to your changing body and growing baby to consume '5 a day' fruit and vegetables. It is something very easy to monitor. If you go for a variety of colours of fruit and vegetables, that will help provide you with a variety of different vitamins and minerals. You could keep a daily chart (maybe on the fridge door) to mark off each time you have one of your 5 a day.

FREQUENT SMALL MEALS ARE BEST

In order to accommodate your growing tummy and restrictions to your digestive area, frequent small meals are easier to manage than two or three large meals each day. This is considered better for your metabolism anyway, so consider following a pattern like this:

- Small carbohydrate and water upon rising to combat nausea
- Breakfast
- Morning snack
- Lunch
- Afternoon snack
- Supper
- Evening snack (a small amount of carbohydrate just before bed can help to alleviate your morning sickness if you are prone to feeling unwell upon waking)
- You may find a middle of the night snack is in order when your baby is going through growth phases. Listen to your body, but try to keep it a healthy snack

Iron during pregnancy is often needed in supplementation form. But an easy way to ensure you get a good intake of iron is through eating an iron-rich breakfast cereal. Iron needs to be teamed with vitamin C in order to help the body absorb it, so fresh (not from concentrate) fruit juice at breakfast is also very important. Likewise, hot drinks may prevent the absorption of iron so are best avoided for an hour before and after eating breakfast.

Eating well does not need to be expensive. A little can go a long way if you shop carefully and cook bulk meals you can freeze. This is a clever practice too for preparing meals for when your baby arrives, as cooking will not be your priority.

CRAVINGS

Cravings are usually your body's way of telling you that you're lacking in something. An extreme example of this is when you hear of pregnant women sucking on lumps of coal – not so much nowadays, more prevalent decades ago. This would have been due to a lack of iron in the diet.

People who crave sweet foods could be in need of more energy. The craving suggests that the consumption of more complex carbohydrates found in wholegrain foods (as these release their energy more slowly throughout the day) would be preferable to consuming simple sugars such as chocolate, which only provide a 'quick fix' and a massive energy crash once you come down from the sugar high.

DID YOU KNOW?

Craving chocolate is often an indication of a lack of certain nutrients such as iron, copper, magnesium and potassium. These nourishing alternatives will help you to replenish your body with these nutrients:

Iron: eat brown rice, whole wheat, dates, beets

Copper: eat nuts (especially cashews), sunflower seeds, chickpeas

Magnesium: eat peanuts, tofu, broccoli, spinach

Potassium: eat apricots, bran wheat, raisins, figs, baked potatoes with skin

---

HOW TO EAT WELL (IF YOU HAVE NO IDEA WHERE TO BEGIN)

We know that some people need a little guidance regarding when and how to eat, so here is an eating plan which you can adapt to the types of food you enjoy. If you are not a plan person, then just ignore this section and follow our 'little and often' motto!

The FitMama™ pregnancy eating plan that follows is an example of one day only; please use your own recipe ideas to add variety to your healthy eating plan, or use some of the healing recipes in chapter 17.

Remember, pregnancy is no time for diets. Your body needs nourishment and hydration. Don't neglect your nutrition by eating too much sugar, or by not eating frequently enough.

If you suffer from any form of eating disorder, please be honest with your midwife so that she can support you throughout your pregnancy. An eating disorder can cover a variety of conditions such as anorexia, bulimia, compulsive overeating or binge eating disorder. If you feel too embarrassed to seek support via your midwife, contact the National Centre for Eating Disorders: www.eating-disorders.org.uk

The FitMama™ pregnancy eating plan

When	Hydration	Food
Upon rising	Warm drink such as redbush (rooibos) tea or warm water and lemon juice	Rice cake or plain tea biscuit to help with feelings of sickness.
Breakfast	Water. If you find water hard to drink alone, add a small amount of organic squash	Complex carbohydrate such as porridge, with fruit; include a spoon of coconut oil* *or* wholemeal toast with poached eggs *or* salmon and avocado.
Mid-morning snack	Water	Take your pick from nuts, fruit, cheese, seeds, vegetable sticks and hummous.

When	Hydration	Food
Lunch	Water	Lean meat or fish with vegetables and brown rice, or salad and brown rice. If you like a sandwich at lunch time, try to eat only wholemeal bread and include plenty of greens and meat/protein choices for the filling.
Mid-afternoon snack	Water	You can revisit the mid-morning snack, but if you're beginning to feel the urge to lie down and sleep, try dates and apricots for a lift. These are also great for pregnancy bowels.
Evening meal	Water	Lean meat or fish and colourful vegetables. Try to avoid starchy foods such as mashed potatoes and pasta as they can aggravate pregnancy heartburn, causing you a difficult night's sleep.
Evening snack	Water. Try to get enough hydration throughout the day so you don't feel too thirsty at night	A little bedtime snack can help combat sugar imbalances in pregnancy, particularly if you suffer from gestational diabetes. Bananas have a sedative effect and can help you sleep through the night. Other options include: small portion of cheese; small serving of oat porridge; tablespoon of peanut butter. *Avoid meats at this time as they can be harder to digest.*

Coconut oil: Raw coconut oil is a medium/short chain saturated fat easily digested, absorbed, and put to use nourishing the body. Unlike other fats, it puts little strain on the digestive system and provides a quick source of energy necessary to promote healing. *Use instead of olive oil or sunflower oils when cooking.*

Some nutritional professionals believe that supplements aren't essential in pregnancy unless recommended by your health carer, as all the nutrients your body needs can be supplied by eating a proper and varied diet. The term 'supplement' means just that: they are to supplement something lacking in your diet, not to be taken as a replacement for something you can get from eating a sensible diet.

You will find a chart outlining which foods will give you essential nutrients to assist the development of your pregnancy, including vitamins and minerals, on pages 21–23.

OBESITY IN PREGNANCY

It is really important to try not to give in to the dangerous sugar cravings you may experience during pregnancy. A treat now and again is not a disaster, but try to ensure your treats are not daily, or more often. Sugar makes bigger babies – ouch!

Sugar hides itself in so called 'healthy' foods, such as energy drinks, fruit juices, yogurts and healthy snack bars, to name a few. Anything man-made and processed is likely to contain hidden sugars.

Normal weight gain during pregnancy is to be expected. By the end of your pregnancy, you should weigh about 12.5 kilograms (27.6 lb) more than you did at the outset. However, if you allow this weight gain to get out of control you will put your skeletal structure at risk. As the pelvis struggles to cope with the ever-evolving pregnant tummy anyway, the added weight you will gain if you lose control of your eating will exacerbate any pregnancy discomfort, put your heart under strain and increase your chances of gestational diabetes, particularly if you are a sugar junkie. Not only this, but you will find your labour and delivery a dangerous challenge as your body has to work with unnecessarily added weight. Extra weight forces your organs to work harder under pressure. You need these to be operating at their optimum during pregnancy and childbirth to ensure your safety.

Obesity in pregnancy is diagnosed when a woman's body mass index (BMI) is measured at 30 and above. Normal BMI in a non-pregnant state is between 20 and 25 for adult women. You can work out your pre-pregnancy BMI using the chart provided opposite. If you are unsure, ask your midwife to help you.

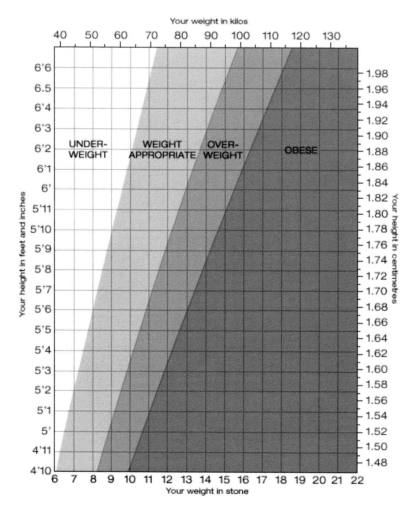

Body Mass Index chart courtesy of National Health
Service Choices www.nhs.uk

If you are worried about your weight and you fall into the obese or very obese category, you are likely to have been given some guidance by your midwife. If not, please do use this chart to assess your healthy pregnancy weight, and if you fall into the overweight or obese zone, please seek advice from your medical practitioner to help you control your pregnancy weight gain.

DID YOU KNOW?

The Royal College of Obstetricians and Gynaecologists found that the prevalence of obesity in the general population in England has increased markedly since the early 1990s. The prevalence of obesity in pregnancy has also been seen to increase, rising from 9-10% in the early 1990s to 16-19% in the 2000s.

Obesity in pregnancy is associated with an increased risk of a number of serious adverse outcomes, including miscarriage, foetal congenital anomaly, thromboembolism, gestational diabetes, pre-eclampsia, dysfunctional labour, postpartum haemorrhage, wound infections, stillbirth and neonatal death.

There is a higher caesarean section rate and lower breast-feeding rate in this group of women compared to women with a healthy BMI. There is also evidence to suggest that obesity may be a risk factor for maternal death: the *Confidential Enquiry into Maternal and Child Health*'s report on maternal deaths in the 2003-2005 triennium showed that 28% of mothers who died were obese, whereas the prevalence of obesity in the general maternity population within the same time period was 16-19%.

You may find some of the facts listed in the above *Did you know?* box upsetting, but knowledge is power, and this is your opportunity to make a difference to your pregnancy. Your maternal weight is in your hands.

I don't believe in a deliberately skinny pregnancy, but I do encourage healthy eating and self-awareness. If you feel you are slipping off the wagon, seek assistance from your midwife to get your eating under control. Ask your family to help you by participating with you. Your health depends on how you manage your sugar intake, and your baby depends on good nutrients to grow and develop well.

You can find more information about eating well during pregnancy on the government 'Eat Well' website: www.eatwell.gov.uk

VITAMINS AND MINERALS

You may be advised to take a vitamin and mineral supplement throughout your pregnancy to help your body achieve optimal health. But if you are not a tablet taker, or would prefer to find your nutritional health through food, this nutritional chart will help you to maximise your nutritional supplementation through good food options.

It is important to bear in mind that overcooking food will impact on the quality of the vitamins and minerals associated with that food group, so try to steam your vegetables rather than boil them. Processed foods will contain preservatives and flavour enhancers which, although they make your food taste nice, are not good for your long-term health, nor that of your baby. Processed foods mean anything which has been put together in a factory, such as ready meals and processed meats.

Although at first you might think so, it is not expensive to shop for fresh food. I find I use less when shopping fresh, which means that I am not throwing out as many leftovers.

Think out of the box, and experiment with putting different types of food together to keep it interesting.

Use the following chart, courtesy of Georgina Wilson, nutritional researcher and former FitMama™ participant, to understand which nutrients help your baby to develop and where to find them.

Nutrient chart

Name	Use	Found in
Vitamin A	Development of baby's bones and teeth, heart, ears, eyes and immune system.	Carrots, sweet potatoes, greens, cantaloupe, eggs, mangos and peas.
Vitamin B6	Helps develop baby's brain and nervous system. Helps both mum and baby develop new red blood cells.	Fortified cereals, bananas, baked potatoes, watermelon, chickpeas and chicken breast.

Name	Use	Found in
Vitamin B12	Works with folic acid to help produce healthy red blood cells and develop the foetal brain and nervous system.	Red meat, poultry, fish, eggs and dairy foods. Vegans can find it in fortified tofu and soya milk.
Vitamin C	Helps body absorb iron and build healthy immune system.	Citrus fruits, raspberries, peppers, green beans, strawberries, broccoli, potatoes and tomatoes.
Calcium	Builds baby's bones and helps brain and heart to function.	Dairy products, fortified juices and cereals, spinach, broccoli, sweet potatoes, lentils, tofu.
Vitamin D	Helps to absorb calcium.	Milk, fortified cereals, eggs, salmon, mackerel. Also in sunshine.
Vitamin E	Helps baby's body to form and also helps baby to use its muscles. Deficiency in mum has been linked to pre-eclampsia.	Vegetable oil, nuts, spinach and fortified cereals.
Folic acid (B9)	Used for the replication of DNA, cell growth and tissue formation – deficiency can lead to neural tube defects.	Oranges, orange juice, strawberries, leafy vegetables, broccoli, cauliflower, peas, pasta, beans and nuts.
Iron	Helps form extra blood and to form the placenta and develop the baby's cells.	Red meat, poultry, legumes, vegetables, some grains and fortified cereals.

Name	Use	Found in
Niacin (B3)	Provides energy for the baby and helps build the placenta.	High protein foods, such as eggs, meats, fish and also whole grains, bread, fortified cereals and milk.
Protein	Growth and development of the baby's body.	Beans, poultry, red meats, fish, eggs, milk, cheese, tofu and yogurts.
Riboflavin (B2)	Development of baby's bones, muscles and nervous system.	Whole grains, dairy products, red meat, pork, poultry, fish, eggs, fortified cereals.
Thiamine (B1)	Helps develop baby's organs and nervous system.	Whole grains, pork, fortified cereals, wheat germ and eggs.
Zinc	Aids cell division.	Red meats, poultry, beans, nuts, grains and dairy products.

CHAPTER 3

Red? Orange? Green? Go!

PHYSIOLOGICAL CHANGES DURING PREGNANCY

Your body will endure some astounding changes during pregnancy, and you may even have been aware of some signs from the very outset. Did you feel suddenly bloated, or perhaps your breasts felt like shards of glass before you even had a positive pregnancy test? You may have felt sick from as early as six days past ovulation. These signs and symptoms were just small signals of the massive changes to come.

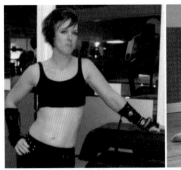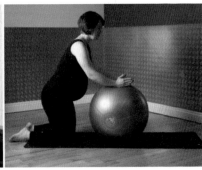

Spot the difference: Left: Our 'rock chick' model Lola, with her sickeningly flat tummy a year before her very convenient pregnancy – just in time for our photo shoot! Right: Lola pregnant at 37 weeks with baby Freddie.

HEART RATE IN PREGNANCY

During pregnancy, blood volume increases by up to 50%. This increase usually takes place between six and 24 weeks gestation. The heart responds to this increase by increasing the heart rate and stroke volume – the amount of blood the heart pumps out. You might have noticed that you become a bit out of breath doing normal things like walking up the stairs, or carrying your shopping to the car. I found this to be one of the earlier signs of my pregnancies. My usual walk to work suddenly felt like an uphill struggle as I panted my way to town.

The pregnant woman will have a higher resting heart rate than during her non-pregnant state, so it is considered that measuring heart rate in pregnancy is not an appropriate form of assessing how much strain exercise is causing the pregnant woman. Instead, it is advised that the more reliable form of assessing breathlessness is by means of the 'talk test'.

If you struggle to talk during exercise or sound breathless, then you are over-exerted for pregnancy. This, coupled with the increased demand on the lungs for oxygen, creating shortness of breath, means you must listen to your body to understand your own limits, and accept that this is a signal to stop.

HOW TO ASSESS WHETHER YOU'RE COPING

It is very easy to assess whether or not you are doing too much. Speaking out loud and completing a whole sentence without gasping for breath is your easiest rule of thumb.

'Talk test' success: You can easily complete a full sentence without gasping for air.

'Talk test' concern: You struggle to catch your breath when talking. Take action and rest.

BLOOD PRESSURE

Due to the change in blood volume during pregnancy there is an effect on blood pressure, which can often be lower than your non-pregnant

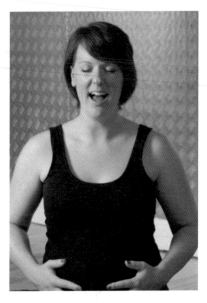

Lola Turvey practises the 'talk test'

reading. This lowering can lead to dizzy spells in early pregnancy. If you feel dizzy when exercising, or when going about your business, this is a good sign to take a rest, drink some water, and put your feet up. If you are under 16 weeks pregnant, elevate your feet above heart level to help your blood pressure find its balance again. If you are over 16 weeks pregnant, lie on your left-hand side (this keeps the vena cava vein clear of pressure) so that your blood can flow easily to your heart and help you feel better. After 16 weeks, avoid lying on your back, so the venous return to the heart is not compromised.

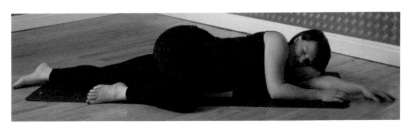

Lola takes a break when feeling dizzy, lying on her left-hand side to free the vena cava and bring her blood pressure back to normal

METABOLISM

During pregnancy, your glucose production will shift carbohydrates to fats more quickly than in your non-pregnant state. This diversion of glucose away from the tissues toward the placenta can lead to a state of ketosis. This, coupled with insulin resistance, necessitates higher calorie intake.

Ketosis happens when the muscles have little, or no, glucose for energy to be able to function efficiently. Once the glucose supply in the bloodstream is depleted, the body starts to break down its fat stores for energy instead. This produces ketones, often causing a fever, body weakness and the muscles – including the uterus – to function inefficiently.

With this higher energy release your body dissipates the excess energy into heat, causing you to feel warmer. This higher body temperature can be harmful to you and your baby. Ensure that you don't overheat during exercise by wearing light, loose clothes, keeping the room well-ventilated and drinking water for hydration.

DID YOU KNOW?

People who have subscribed to particular diets, such as the Palaeolithic (caveman) diet, strive to attain ketosis. The pregnant woman needs to understand the dangers of this state of metabolism to safeguard her and her baby. It is important for her to remain well-hydrated and to eat a balanced diet which includes carbohydrates.

POSTURE

From the outset of pregnancy one thing is certain: the baby will grow, and your posture will bear the brunt of this growth. As the baby grows, the pelvis will tilt forward. This can happen on one side or both, in equal or unbalanced proportions. This will impact on the lower back, and in many cases the knees will lock. The knock-on effect can display itself in the shoulder girdle posture, a slouch, as the head is carried forward, taking ears out of alignment with shoulders. Ribs can flare out, particularly in the case of hyper-mobile women (see overleaf).

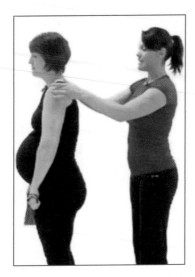

Marie teaches Lola how to correct her posture during pregnancy.
Note Lola's rounded shoulders and sway back, caused by the
excess burden of the abdominal changes

RELAXIN

Aches and pains are common in pregnancy, thanks to relaxin. Relaxin is produced by the corpus luteum (what is left of the follicle after a woman ovulates), myometrium (the smooth muscle tissue of the uterus), and the placenta.

Relaxin has a role in softening the elastic ligaments of pelvic bones in preparation for birth. But relaxin is not specific to the pelvic bones and so other joints are affected, which can cause great discomfort to you during pregnancy. For example, some women find their wrists are very painful, so hand and knee positions can be unbearable for them.

You may experience pelvic girdle pain (formerly known as symphesis pubis dysfunction and sacroiliac joint dysfunction) in pregnancy, associated with the stretching of pelvic girdle ligaments. You may feel this posterior pain as lower back ache. This discomfort is greatly aided by working on pelvic stability through a variety of exercises specific to pelvic girdle support.

Relaxin can also cause a flare-up of old injuries sustained well before pregnancy.

HYPER-MOBILITY

Hyper-mobility describes joints that stretch further than is normal for joint stability. For example, some hyper-mobile people can bend their thumbs backwards to their wrists, bend their knee joints backwards, and put their leg behind the head or other contortionist performances. It can affect a single joint or multiple joints throughout the body. In pregnancy, women with joint hyper-mobility, or conditions such as Marfan syndrome or Ehlers-Danlos syndrome (see below), may be at increased risk of pelvic organ prolapse. This is where the organs inside the pelvis slip down from their normal position. For example, the uterus (womb) may slip down into the vagina.

If you suffer from these conditions or a pre-existing abdominal hernia you will need to take extra care in strengthening the support groups of muscles to aid stability in the joints, and you are advised to ask for physiotherapist support via your midwife before attempting the exercises in this book.

DID YOU KNOW?

Marfan syndrome is a disorder of connective tissue, the tissue that strengthens the body's structures. Disorders of connective tissue affect the skeletal system, cardiovascular system, eyes and skin.

Ehlers-Danlos syndrome is a group of inherited disorders marked by extremely loose joints, hyper-elastic skin that bruises easily, and easily damaged blood vessels.

GETTING STARTED

If you are healthy, well and have not suffered any adverse complications, I want you to be active, mobile and find a good balance between exercise and rest throughout your pregnancy. But before you begin any exercise routine during pregnancy, you must follow the guidelines to ensure you are not putting yourself at risk:

- Ensure that you are feeling well and are not suffering any contraindicated symptoms of pregnancy (see page 32).

- Ensure that your midwife or medical care-giver is aware that you plan to exercise during your pregnancy, and discuss any concerns that you may have with them.
- Always ensure that your exercise environment is safe, well-ventilated and that the room temperature is cool. Your body temperature will rise during exercise, so never exercise in a warm room; 18°C (65°F) is about right.
- Always ensure you have enough water available to keep yourself hydrated. Dehydration is extremely dangerous at any time of your life, let alone pregnancy.
- Ensure that you are wearing comfortable clothes. Don't forget a supportive bra to support the Coopers ligaments (connective tissue) of your growing pregnancy breasts (this will protect you from long-term damage and save you from droopy boobs)!
- Ensure you wear safe footwear, or are barefoot on a safe surface if you can't get your trainers on these days. Don't exercise in socks as you could slip and injure yourself.

DEHYDRATION DURING PREGNANCY

Dehydration occurs when your body eliminates more water than you take in. This means you are not drinking enough water and your body actually dries out. Dehydration is a major contributor to such heat illnesses as heat cramps, heat exhaustion and heat stroke. Dehydration can become a risk to your pregnancy health very quickly.

In the early stages of pregnancy, being dehydrated (usually caused by morning sickness) can cause nausea, creating a cycle because your nausea stops you from wanting to drink anything, and therefore you become more nauseous, in turn becoming more dehydrated, which can feel distressing and raise your stress levels. This can result in hospitalisation overnight for intravenous fluids.

Dehydration in the first trimester and part of the second can impact on the levels of amniotic fluid for your baby – a significant lack of amniotic fluid can cause the baby to lie against the uterus rather than float in the amniotic fluid, which may cause deformities of the limbs. During the second and third trimesters, dehydration is one of the common causes of premature labour.

Dehydration is known to raise your body temperature, which might lead to further complications, such as cramping and heat exhaustion. Finally, dehydration can exacerbate fatigue during pregnancy.

It is not always obvious to us that we are dehydrated, so it may help you to keep an eye out for signs that you are:

- Thirst. This is the first sign, and is often confused with thinking you are a bit hungry. If you find you are looking in the fridge for a snack but don't actually feel hungry, have a glass of water as you will no doubt be dehydrated. Listen to your body – if you feel thirsty, your body is trying to tell you something. Try to keep a bottle of water with you all the time so you can take sips regularly through the day.
- Lightheaded or dizzy feelings, especially when standing up, bending over, or kneeling. Low blood pressure caused by dehydration will make you feel like this. Sit down and drink water.
- Headaches, including migraines.
- Dark yellow urine (your vitamins can cause this too, but dehydration will cause your urine to smell potent).
- Lack of regular urination.
- Dry mouth and nose, and chapped lips.
- Muscular weakness.
- Nausea and vomiting.
- Skin can become excessively dry.

The best prevention and cure for dehydration is drinking water. If the body doesn't have enough water your major organs and those of your baby will not function properly. During exercise, or any situation where your body temperature will become raised, such as in the summer or in a well-heated room, you are likely to become dehydrated without realising.

Some drinks are dehydrating, such as caffeine, which is found in coffee, tea, fizzy drinks and fruit juice made from concentrate. If you don't like plain water, try adding a little squash or a slice of lemon to the water.

If you are going to travel by air during your pregnancy, keep water with you, as the dry air in the cabin is dehydrating.

You are advised to ask your midwife or GP how much water you should be taking on a daily basis during your pregnancy, and seek advice if you suspect you are suffering from severe dehydration.

CONTRAINDICATIONS FOR EXERCISE DURING PREGNANCY

There are some cases where pregnancy can mean specific prescribed exercise only, or in some cases no exercise at all. If you are prescribed specific exercise due to some health concerns, you are considered to fall into the *relative contraindications* category.

In this category, you are advised to exercise caution and to discuss with your medical professional how your exercise programme should be approached and what to avoid. If you have any of the following, or if any of the following applies to you, only proceed with an exercise programme under supervision of your healthcare provider and qualified prenatal fitness professional (ACOG guidelines):

- Heart problems, high blood pressure/hypertension, or maternal cardio arrhythmia
- Anaemia
- Asthma, chronic bronchitis or lung problems
- Diabetes
- Thyroid problems
- Seizures
- Extreme over- or under- weight
- Muscle or joint problems
- History of spontaneous miscarriages
- History of previous premature labour
- Carrying multiple babies (eg twins, triplets)
- A previously sedentary lifestyle
- Smoking (I absolutely recommend that you quit smoking during pregnancy; if you can't by yourself, visit your midwife for advice)
- Orthopaedic limitations
- Intrauterine growth restriction in current pregnancy

> The Guild of Pregnancy and Postnatal Exercise Instructors will have a list of suitable professionals in your area. www.postnatal exercise.co.uk

If you are prescribed no exercise due to health concerns, you fall into the *absolute contraindications* category. In this category of conditions, you are advised that you should not participate in an exercise programme during pregnancy (ACOG guidelines):

- Haemodynamically significant heart disease
- Restrictive lung disease
- Incompetent cervix or cerclage (a procedure where the cervix is sewn closed during pregnancy)
- Multiple pregnancy with babies at risk of premature labour
- Persistent second or third trimester bleeding
- Placenta previa after 28 weeks of gestation (placenta is attached to the uterine wall close to or covering the cervix)
- Premature labour during current pregnancy
- Ruptured membranes (a term used to describe waters breaking)
- Pre-eclampsia, also called pregnancy-induced hypertension. (This condition typically starts after the 20th week of pregnancy and is related to increased blood pressure and protein in the mother's urine. Pre-eclampsia affects the placenta, and it can affect the mother's kidney, liver and brain. The solution to this condition is to deliver the baby to secure both the mother's and the baby's health)

It is vital for your health and the safety of your baby that you listen to the recommendations should you fall into any of these two categories. Your wellbeing and that of your baby is your primary concern. Even if you cannot exercise, you can still arm yourself with the educational knowledge about pelvic floor work, breathing and gentle movement for labour.

WARNING SIGNS: WHEN TO STOP EXERCISING AND CALL YOUR DOCTOR

If you have been well during your pregnancy and you experience anything untoward during exercise, you must cease exercise immediately. If you experience any of the following symptoms, stop exercising and call your health provider right away:

- Bleeding from your vagina
- Difficult breathing/breathlessness before you exercise
- Dizziness
- Headache
- Chest pains
- Muscle weakness
- Calf pain or swelling
- Preterm labour
- Leakage of amniotic fluid from your vagina
- Contractions of your uterus
- Feeling your baby move significantly less inside

Call your doctor *immediately* if you have any of these symptoms.

(Source: American College of Obstetricians and Gynecologists, *Exercise during pregnancy and the postpartum period,* Obstetrics & Gynecology, volume 99, number 1, January 2002, pages 171–173.)

The exercise techniques

Preface to the exercises

The following exercises are designed for you to perform safely on your own, and so you will only find exercises that work you in a safe plane of movement direction. I will presume that you are suffering from pelvic discomfort; this will act to ensure your safety and prevent you from doing damage to your softening ligaments as your pregnancy progresses.

My method offers exercises suitable for all stages of your pregnancy, which is why you won't see sections for each trimester: you are only ever practising exercise suitable for your most sensitive stages of pregnancy.

My method tries to train you out of bad habits right from the outset. That means you will never lie on your back for any of these pregnancy exercises, to keep your arteries free from the pressure of the weight of the baby when in this position.

You will not find a sit-up or abdominal crunch in this programme, not least because they are completely pointless exercises and not considered safe for the pregnant woman. If you are in the early (pre-16 week) phase of your pregnancy and you are doing this type of exercise in any group classes you attend, you can continue until 16 weeks, but please let your instructor know when you are nearing 16 weeks so that suitable alternatives can be offered to you. If your instructor does not have a prenatal qualification, please consider finding one who is qualified to advise you during your sessions.

The FitMama™ method of exercises is aimed at women from all fitness backgrounds. Women who have never exercised before can use it as a gentle introduction and maintenance plan for pregnancy. Women who are more athletic and find it difficult to take it easy can

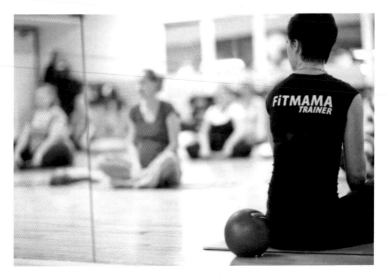

FitMama™ exercise class: pelvic floor training

use this method as a grounding approach for a pregnancy exercise programme – a means to find a less intensive form of mobility and maintenance.

Most importantly, this programme is about keeping you mobile, flexible, safe and self-aware. Enjoy it, and find the level that is right for you within the method.

HOW PREGNANT DO I NEED TO BE?

You can begin this programme at any stage, as long as you are well and healthy and do not identify with any of the contraindications set out in chapter 3. The exercises can be executed at the level you feel comfortable with, so you can adapt them to how you feel.

If you are new to exercise, do as much as you can without exhausting yourself. If you are experienced at exercise, do the whole programme – but listen to your body on your off days!

EQUIPMENT

Although fitness balls, Pilates balls and resistance bands are used in these exercises, they are not a prerequisite. You can use items from around the house to help: for instance, sit on a chair instead of a ball; hold cans of beans instead of a resistance band. Be creative!

If you are using a real fitness ball, please ensure it is correctly inflated and that you have purchased the correct size for your height:

45cm ball: suitable for height 5'0" (152cm) or shorter
55cm ball: suitable for height 5'1" – 5'6" (155cm – 167cm)
65cm ball: suitable for height 5'7" – 6'1" (170cm – 185cm)
75cm ball: suitable for height 6'2" (188cm) or taller

PELVIC FLOOR SQUEEZE

You will read the phrase 'keep your pelvic floor tidy' in this book. This means that you need to squeeze your bladder and back passage as though you need to go to the toilet. Don't squeeze hard, just a gentle squeeze – as though you only need to go to the toilet in a few moments, not with urgency. This is a quick and easy way to engage the pelvic floor group of muscles so that you can train them effectively throughout your pregnancy.

To ensure that you understand how to engage these muscles, you can test that this pelvic floor squeeze works when you next visit the toilet by simply stopping the flow of urine while you empty your bladder. But please do not use this test as an exercise; you would be in danger of causing a urinary tract infection if you did this on a regular basis.

HOW OFTEN SHOULD I FOLLOW THE EXERCISE ROUTINE?

I would like you to try to achieve an exercise from each section of the book three times each week. For example, on day 1, choose perhaps 5 exercises. Do each exercise for 8 repetitions times 3 sets, including both arms and legs if relevant. On day 2, choose 7 exercises for 8 repetitions times 3 sets; on day 3, choose less or more, depending on how you feel. (An example of 8 repetitions times 3 sets: do 8 squats;

have a little rest; do another 8 squats; rest; do the final 8 squats.) If you are feeling energetic and can manage all of the exercises every day without exhausting yourself, that is great. Remember to listen to your body. If you are too tired, perhaps just a gentle walk to rebalance your energy levels is the answer. If you are feeling energetic and well, try the whole programme.

Your body will always tell you what you feel up to undertaking.

CHAPTER 4

It's all in the heart

I am amazed by how many people do not realise the level of fitness required to push your baby out. Earlier in the book I likened the process of labour and delivery to running a marathon. I was not exaggerating! The amount of pressure your heart will be put under during labour is the same as the amount of pressure you would feel when running great distances.

Labour and delivery represent considerable effort for pregnant women. Low aerobic (heart/respiratory) fitness may limit pushing efforts during childbirth and represents increased cardiovascular strain and risk.

Fortunately, labour has a degree of interval training to it. This means that the intensity ebbs and flows, so you will have moments of rest between moments of intense contracting and pushing. The only way to ensure that your heart can handle this is to make sure you keep it well trained during your pregnancy. If the heart is kept fit and well, you can bet that during labour it will cope extremely well and will help you to have a very positive delivery experience.

APPROPRIATE EXERCISE

As you know, the heart will undertake extra work during pregnancy. Blood volume increases by up to 50% and the heart responds by increasing the heart rate and stroke volume (the amount of blood the heart pumps out). So, how do you think you can get your heart finely tuned for a successful attempt at natural delivery?

If you have been attending energetic aerobic-style fitness classes regularly up to the time you conceived, you can continue at the level you are used to. Many people make the mistake of thinking they need to stop their usual exercise and spend more time with their feet up. By now, if you are not suffering from any contraindications mentioned earlier in the book, you will know how I feel about that! The rule for a healthy pregnancy is that you can continue with the exercise you are used to. Your body will tell you when it's too much for you to cope with. How? Well, you just won't find it as easy as you used to, or you might not even feel like attending at all. Of course, if you begin to experience pain, bleeding, or any other unpleasant symptoms, this is a sign to cease these classes and seek advice about suitable prenatal exercise in your area.

If your cardio exercise has always taken the form of horse riding, you may find as you become more pregnant that your safety on the horse is compromised by your changing centre of gravity. I would advise you seek an alternative to this exercise. The same applies if you participate in any contact sport, for example kickboxing or rugby, which could compromise the safety of your baby.

THE GREAT OUTDOORS

So, what if you are not a member of the gym? Well, in my opinion there is nothing better than the great outdoors to invigorate a pregnant body. In particular, if you have never exercised before you can take advantage of nature. Walking is a highly underrated form of exercise. The best things about walking are that you can do it at your own pace and you can easily incorporate it into your everyday life.

You may wonder how you can make your heart fit just by walking. I love hill walking! Using powerful strides up a steep hill is a brilliant way to increase heart fitness and prepare your heart for the challenge of labour. The great news about walking outdoors is that the terrain will create the natural interval training you need to prepare your heart for labour. Try to find a route with some uphill stretches, some downhill stretches and some flat roads.

These are my top tips for safe pregnancy walking to improve your fitness for labour:

1. Wear safe shoes for walking – trainers or hiking shoes – and ensure you are not wearing clothes in which you will overheat. Light layers are best so you can manage your heat levels by taking off a layer as you get warmer.
2. Ensure you have water with you for hydration; sip little amounts to avoid getting a stitch.
3. Try to walk tall and keep your baby tucked in using your natural tummy strength (see the pelvic floor section to understand more about this).
4. Try to walk with your heels touching the ground first and then massage the rest of the foot into the stride until the toes leave the ground. Keep your arms moving with the rhythm of your walk.
5. When walking up hills, try to power up the hill using your gluteals (bottom cheeks), and ensure you don't overexert yourself.
6. Remember to do the 'talk test' (see page 25) whilst walking; you could recite a phrase to yourself to ensure you are able to talk without losing your breath, for instance 'The fit pregnant lady walked up the steep green hill'. If you cannot complete the phrase, this is a clear sign you need to stop walking and recover!
7. If you feel a stitch in your side when you are walking, slow your pace, come to a rest and take in some water. Side stitches are thought to be caused by dehydration.
8. If you experience any of the following, you must stop and call for help:

    * Persistent or unusual headaches
    * Persistent nausea and vomiting
    * Dizziness
    * Disturbances of eyesight
    * Pain or cramps in the lower abdomen
    * Contractions
    * Vaginal bleeding
    * Leakage of amniotic fluid (waters break)
    * Swelling of the hands or feet
    * Decreased urine production
    * Any illness or feelings of infection (feeling feverish)

- Tremor (shaking of the hands, feet, or both)
- Seizures
- Rapid heart rate
- Decreased movement of the foetus

9. Try not to walk in isolated areas in case you become unwell during your walk and need assistance.
10. Ensure you have a mobile phone with you in case you become overwhelmed and need to call on a friend to come and drive you home.
11. If you wear headphones to listen to music while you exercise, keep one ear free so that you can hear traffic and goings on around you.
12. Breathe! You would be surprised how many people hold their breath during exercise. Take great care to inhale and exhale as you walk. As you exhale, the oxygen makes the exchange from the lungs into the bloodstream, taking the energy to your muscles and organs. If you hold your breath, you will starve your body of the air you need to exercise.

HOW OFTEN SHOULD YOU BE WALKING?

I recommend that you try to factor walking into your daily life. For example, if you are working through your pregnancy, take 20 minutes during your lunch break to go for a brisk walk, and complete your session with something to eat and a drink to keep you going through the afternoon. If you are at home with children, try to take them for walks with you and make it a bonding time together.

Don't forget to eat and drink regularly throughout the day. When you are at home and busy with children, you tend to feed them and forget yourself, or just pick at what you've served the children. Try to get into the habit of refuelling after exercise.

HOW LONG SHOULD YOU BE WALKING FOR?

Twenty to 30 minutes of walking for each session is about the time you should aim for during pregnancy. However, you should listen to your body, and if you can only manage 10 minutes, then 10 minutes is good enough! In some cases less is more. There is no point in exhausting yourself; exercise should be energising, not draining, on the pregnant body.

If you know other pregnant or postnatal mums, you could arrange a weekly gathering where you walk together and encourage each other to keep active and share experiences.

Remember, your heart fitness is key to your ability to endure the length and intensity of your labour. A healthy heart will help you cope more effectively!

CHAPTER 5

Pregnant and bootylicious!

We all want a pert bottom, but in some cases women resign themselves to the fact that with pregnancy comes a big bottom. Well, if you sit on your bottom and eat cakes all day, yes, that is true. There is a degree of body fat being laid down in preparation for breastfeeding when the baby is born, but with good nutrition and exercise your bottom should not end up being massively bigger than when you entered your pregnancy.

But I'm not really interested in the aesthetics of pregnancy bottoms! I'm much more interested in how the bottom can help your pregnancy as it develops and grows.

The muscles of the bottom and legs go a long way to help stabilise our skeletal structure. This is important because as a baby grows inside us, the added weight of the baby, placenta and fluids weighs heavily on the pelvis, forcing it out of its neutral position. In turn, the posture of the spine can be thrown out of alignment and cause us great discomfort.

In the picture on page 28, you can see that Lola is displaying the sway back of pregnancy, where her spine has taken on an 'S' shape, adding pressure to the pelvis, spine and shoulder girdle. You can see how her pregnant tummy almost appears to pull her spine out of alignment and tilt her pelvis. Her ligaments (which hold the bones, cartilage and joints together) are swimming in the relaxin hormone which relaxes the intrauterine ligaments. Your body needs flexibility to enable the uterus and pelvis to accommodate your baby, who will grow from a pin prick to the size of a small watermelon.

I encourage you to keep the muscles of your bottom and legs

strong to help stabilise the pelvis. This will go a long way towards easing the lower back ache often associated with pregnancy. Not only does keeping these muscles strong help your comfort and posture during pregnancy, but if you choose to be upright during labour you will definitely need muscle tone to help support you in this position.

Traditionally, squats and lunges are the best exercises for training legs and bottoms, but during pregnancy you may find lunges uncomfortable to do, particularly if you are suffering from any pubic pain associated with ligament softening. On this basis, I prefer to train pregnant women in simpler planes of motion to help lessen any possibility of aggravating ligament problems.

Keep your posture safe with these basic leg strengthening exercises. You can do them barefoot, as long as the floor surface is safe. Alternatively, wear trainers if you prefer to have the stability of an exercise shoe.

THE FITMAMA™ LEG TRAINING SESSION

In this training session for legs, I have used a gym ball to help Lola stay upright and reduce pressure in the lower back. However, if you do not have a gym ball, you can simply squat without one, and if you prefer the support of a wall behind you, then slide against the wall.

Your feet should not be wider apart than the width of your shoulders; your toes should be pointing out in front of you. Avoid putting your feet into a ballerina position or duck-feet position as this takes the joints out of alignment and can agitate ligaments, which will cause you pain.

When squatting, avoid going deeper than a 90-degree angle at the knee as this puts too much pressure on the joints. If you feel pain in your knees or lower back you are probably going too deep. Try performing a small squat instead. If you still experience pain, avoid this exercise.

The following exercises will help you if you wish to be in an upright position during your labour and delivery time. Upright positions enable the descent of your baby more effectively. Strong legs will help you maintain the position for longer periods of time.

GYM BALL SQUAT

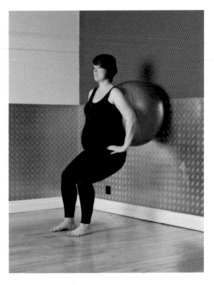

Gym ball squat

Prepare
Lean against the gym ball so that you can see your toes.
Inhale.
Exhale as you zip up your pelvic floor by tidying up your bladder and back passage.

Perform the exercise
Inhale.
Exhale as you sit down into your squat position.
Don't go too deep, as this will compromise your lower back.
If you experience back pain doing this, try to do half the distance in the squat.

Repetitions
8 repetitions × 3 sets

Breathing and pace
Try to move at the pace of your breathing. It is essential to use your full exhalation on the journey down into the squat. Inhale to return to standing.

Adaptations
You can also perform this exercise with a small soft ball held between your thighs. This can serve to help with any discomfort in the pubic bone, or simply keep your knees from pushing out to the side as you sit. It will also help to activate the inner thigh muscles, which in turn will help the pelvic floor muscles to activate, creating an all-round stabilising workout for the pregnant pelvis.

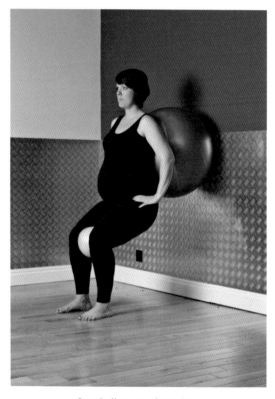

Gym ball squat adaptation

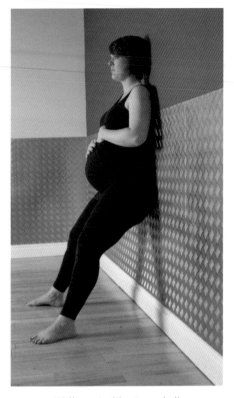

Wall squat without gym ball

Above, Lola demonstrates the wall squat without a gym ball. Lola is strong enough to perform this exercise with a distance between her feet, but if your pelvis is hurting remember to put a ball or cushion between your thighs for stabilisation and pain reduction. Baby Freddy looks like he's getting a mummy cuddle during this exercise!

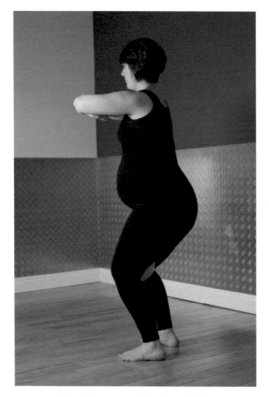

Standing squat without gym ball

You can try standing squats without the support of the gym ball. Ensure you do not sit too deep into this position as you need to keep your spine long and safe. The soft ball held between the thighs activates the inner thighs and pelvic floor groups of muscles, creating stability.

CALF RAISES

You need strong calf muscles to support and stabilise the knee joints. Knee pain is a common affliction during pregnancy, and you can comfort this pain by keeping your lower leg muscles in good condition.

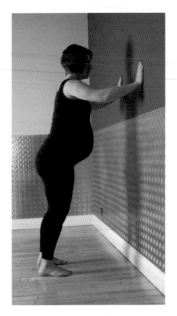

Prepare for calf raise

Prepare
Lean against wall with your hands about shoulder distance apart.
Inhale.
Exhale as you zip up your pelvic floor by tidying up your bladder and back passage.

Perform the exercise
Inhale.
Exhale as you elevate your heels away from the floor.
You may feel cramping in your calves if you are dehydrated, so stop and take in some water if you do.

Repetitions
8 repetitions × 3 sets

Breathing and pace
Try to move at the pace of your breathing. It is essential to use your full exhalation on the journey up onto your toes. Inhale to return to heels down.

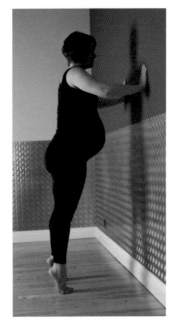

Perform calf raise

CHAPTER 6

Chest out, shoulders back!

In the last chapter I mentioned the 'S' shape of the spine in relation to posture. The shoulder girdle, a group of bones that supports the muscles and ligaments of the shoulders, is often already a weak area in women when they enter pregnancy. You can tell if this is the case if you slouch more often than not. Tight chest muscles do not help either, as they shorten the muscles to the front of the shoulder girdle, forcing your shoulders to slump forward.

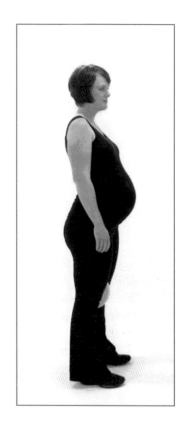

Have a look at Lola's example of the slouch in the shoulder girdle area. Women often develop this stance from their teenage years. Teenage girls can be self-conscious of their developing breasts, and so create the slouch look in an attempt to hide this sudden arrival into womanhood. Sometimes we are not even aware that we have this posture, so it is a good idea to stand sideways on to the mirror and have a look to see if you are slouching.

It is important to take care of your posture, as poor posture can cause a variety of aches and pains, can lower self-esteem and make you feel larger than you really are. When your baby is born, you will need good posture and shoulder strength to help you cope with carrying your baby, breastfeeding or bottle feeding for long periods of time, and all the general multi-tasking you will be doing as a new mum.

If you already have children, you will be familiar with this scenario: holding the baby whilst answering the phone and stirring what you have cooking on the stove. True multi-tasking motherhood style! But not easy to do if your muscles are weak through the shoulder girdle.

By following the basic upper postural exercises in this chapter, you can remove your slouch and strengthen your shoulder girdle. This will improve your natural posture, which will have a positive effect on the natural activation of your pelvic floor muscles. Your organs will function more effectively, and you will generally feel better about yourself.

THE FITMAMA™ SHOULDER GIRDLE AND UPPER BODY TRAINING SESSION

You can sit on a chair for this training session for the shoulder girdle and upper back. But sitting on a gym ball is considered to be a more naturally neutral position, and takes the strain off your back. It also creates a level of instability so that your tummy muscles have to work a bit harder to keep you upright. If you find that you cannot balance safely on a gym ball, please take the more stable option of sitting on a chair.

These exercises use a resistance band. Buy one, or improvise with household objects.

Remember, your safety is of highest importance. So please ensure there are not sharp objects, such as corners of coffee tables, near you in the exercise area. Also ensure the floor is clear of other exercise equipment, or toys if there are children in the house.

GYM BALL SEATED SHOULDER RETRACTION

Prepare

Sit on a chair or gym ball.

Exhale as you zip up your pelvic floor by tidying up your bladder and back passage.

Keep your spine long and tall.

Extend your arms out, holding the resistance band with your hands shoulder distance apart.

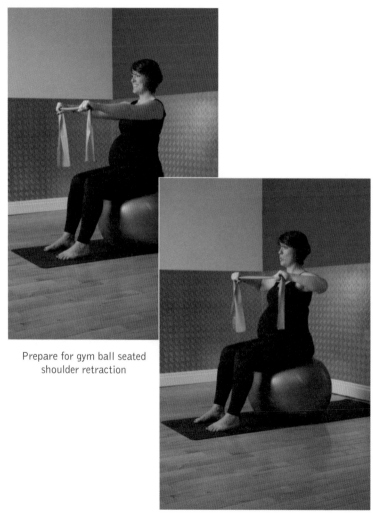

Prepare for gym ball seated
shoulder retraction

Perform gym ball seated
shoulder retraction

Perform the exercise
Inhale.
Exhale as you draw your hands back and your elbows move in the direction of your back.
Stop when your elbows line up with your shoulders.
Inhale and return to the start position.
Try to keep your pelvic floor zipped up during the whole movement.

Repetitions
8 repetitions × 3 sets

Breathing and pace
Try to move at the pace of your breathing. It is essential to use your full exhalation through the movement.

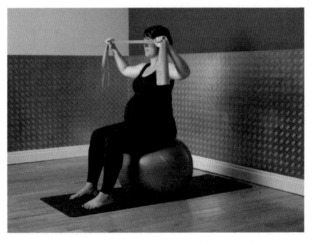

Progression of gym ball seated shoulder retraction

Progression
You can add to this exercise if you feel ready.
At the point of retraction, when your elbows are lined up with your shoulders, you can rotate the band up toward your eyebrow line. This will activate the small muscles of your shoulder cap to give you a more effective exercise for your upper body.

SEATED TRICEPS EXTENSIONS

Triceps are an often-neglected group of muscles at the back of the arms. Once your baby is born, triceps are important to enable you to carry your baby whilst maintaining excellent posture. Get ahead of the game and start training them now. If your triceps are weak you will struggle to carry your baby for long periods, and you'll find that your posture is affected, and the slouch tends to return.

The following exercises involve the use of weights. If you don't have any, use household objects such as tins of baked beans.

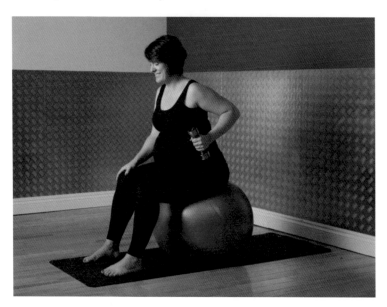

Prepare for seated triceps extensions

Prepare

Sit on a chair or gym ball.

Exhale as you zip up your pelvic floor by tidying up your bladder and back passage.

Tip slightly forward, as much as your growing baby will allow.

Keep your spine long.

Bend your arm at the elbow, and lift your elbow so your hand is close to your ribs.

Keep your feet hip-distance apart for stability.

Perform the exercise
Inhale.
Exhale as you extend your hand and the weight behind you.
Stop when your hand lines up with your elbow.
Inhale and return to the start position.
Try to keep your pelvic floor zipped up during the whole movement.
Do not swing your shoulder; this movement comes from the elbow.

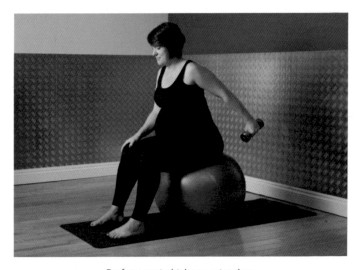

Perform seated triceps extensions

Repetitions
8 repetitions × 3 sets, each arm!

Breathing and pace
Try to move at the pace of your breathing. It is essential to use your full exhalation through the movement.

Adaptation
If you feel strong enough, you could try doing both arms at the same time. Keep your baby tidy with your tummy muscles, as both arms may be more of a challenge and you may find that you forget about your pelvic floor and core muscles.

SHOULDER BUTTERFLIES

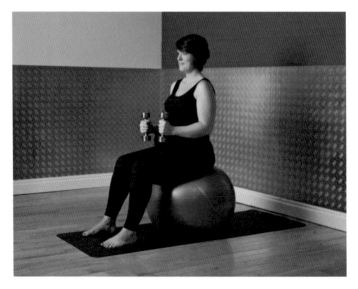

Prepare for shoulder butterflies

Prepare

Using light weights, sit on a chair or gym ball.

Exhale as you zip up your pelvic floor by tidying up your bladder and back passage.

Keep your spine long and tall.

Bend your arm at the elbow, and line your elbow up under your shoulder with your hands to the front of you.

Keep your feet hip-distance apart for stability.

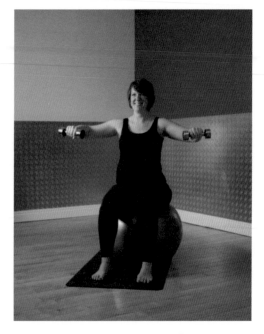

Perform shoulder butterflies

Perform the exercise
Inhale.
Exhale as you elevate your elbows and hands up towards your shoulders.
Stop when your elbows and hands are the same alignment as your
shoulders.
Inhale and return to the start position.

Repetitions
8 repetitions × 3 sets, or the same for each arm if you prefer to do
one arm at a time.

Breathing and pace
Try to move at the pace of your breathing. It is essential to use your
full exhalation through the movement. Try to keep your pelvic floor
zipped up during the whole movement. Try not to slouch during this
exercise. The movement comes from the shoulder.

CHEST PRESS WITH RESISTANCE BAND ON GYM BALL

As your breasts become heavier with the progression of your pregnancy, you will need to ensure that their muscles are working well enough to support the Cooper's ligaments. Always wear a supportive bra to help combat the excess weight of pregnant breasts.

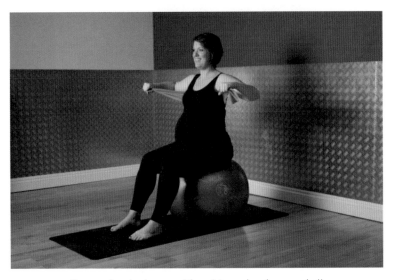

Prepare for chest press with resistance band on gym ball

Prepare

Sit on a chair or gym ball.

Place the resistance band around your back, under your arms and hold the ends in each hand.

Exhale as you zip up your pelvic floor by tidying up your bladder and back passage.

Keep your spine long.

Bend your arms at the elbow, and lift your elbows so that your hands are lined up with your shoulders.

Keep your feet hip-distance apart for stability.

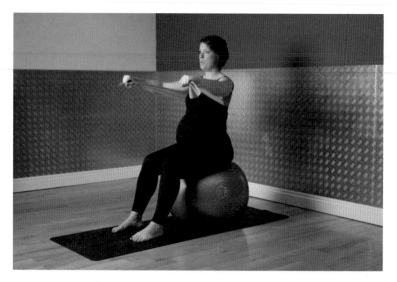

Perform chest press with resistance band on gym ball

Perform the exercise
Inhale.
Exhale as you push your hands forward.
Stop when your arms are fully extended, with a soft elbow.
Inhale and return to the start position.
Try to keep your pelvic floor zipped up during the whole movement.
Do not hunch the shoulders up to the ears.

Repetitions
8 repetitions × 3 sets

Breathing and pace
Try to move at the pace of your breathing. It is essential to use your full exhalation through the movement.

SEATED ROWS

Your upper back will benefit from these rowing movements. Your focus needs to be on trying to get the bones of the shoulder blades to touch each other. If you struggle to sit upright in the specified position, place a cushion under your bottom or wedge a soft ball behind your hips to help tilt your pelvis forward for ease of upright sitting.

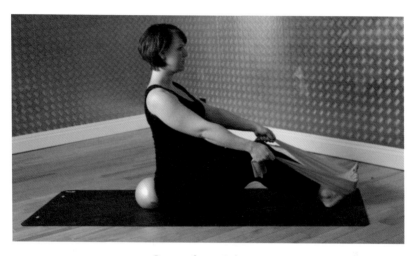

Prepare for seated rows

Prepare
Sit on the floor with your feet out in front of you. Bend your knees. Place the resistance band around the soles of your feet and hold the ends in each hand.
Exhale as you zip up your pelvic floor by tidying up your bladder and back passage.
Keep your spine long and tall.
Lengthen your arms, keeping a soft elbow.

Perform the exercise
Inhale.
Exhale as you draw your elbows behind you.
Stop when feel the squeeze as your shoulder blades (the bones at the back of your shoulders) come together.
Inhale and return to the start position.
Try to keep your pelvic floor zipped up during the whole movement.

Repetitions
8 repetitions × 3 sets

Breathing and pace
Try to move at the pace of your breathing. It is essential to use your full exhalation through the movement. Do not slouch in this position.

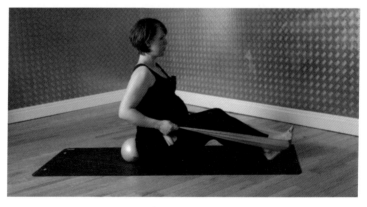

Perform seated rows

Note: You may notice that in this chapter I have not covered bicep training (biceps are the muscles at the front of your upper arms). This is because, in my opinion, we tend to overuse our biceps in daily life, such as when we carry shopping bags, pick up our children, put heavy items into the boot of the car, etc. I would prefer you to focus on your triceps exercises to facilitate bicep ability and improve your posture.

CHAPTER 7

Are you resting your tea on your bump yet?

Let's face it, the first thing to relax when you find out you're pregnant is your tummy! Most women will admit that they see the pregnancy test result and think 'Phew, I don't have to hold my tummy in now!' As comforting a thought as this might be, it is the worst thing you can do for your core strength and posture. You need to keep your abdominal muscles toned, cared for and working hard to support your changing shape and protect you from misalignment of posture.

I do not recommend traditional sit-ups and crunches at any time in life, let alone pregnancy. They are one-dimensional exercises which generally lead to neck ache and other problems. You are better off without them.

Instead, I have put together a selection of exercises which will be more useful to you in pregnancy and will mimic the action of delivery to help prepare your body for this event.

The muscles of the abdomen are very important during delivery. They will work with your contractions to help push your baby towards the birth canal and into the big wide world. In particular, the oblique muscles (muscles which form the shape of your waistline) will be directly involved in the contraction process during labour and delivery. The contractions will create a rippling effect of the muscles in a downward motion, directing the baby towards the exit. The more tuned-in you are to your abdominal strength, the more confident you will be with your pushing. We will discuss pushing techniques later in the book.

If you have planned a caesarean section, you may think 'Well, I don't need to do these exercises!' Please do still do them! They will aid your recovery from the pregnancy and caesarean procedure, and give your muscles the strength to return to a non-pregnant state.

THE FITMAMA™ CORE STABILITY SESSION

THE STANDING PELVIC TILT

This exercise is essential for creating strength through the pelvic floor, but also helps you to practise shortening your long tummy muscles in preparation for pushing out your baby.

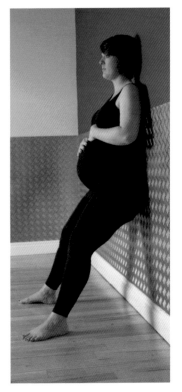

Prepare
Stand with your spine against the wall, feet no wider apart than the width of your pelvis.

Perform the exercise
Inhale.
Exhale as you tilt your pelvis away from the wall, pressing your back into the wall.
Tidy up the pelvic floor as you tilt.
Inhale to return to the start point.

Repetitions
5–10 repetitions

Adaptation
Try this seated on the gym ball.

The standing pelvic tilt

THE CORE CAT

This exercise can be executed safely on your hands and knees. Note that Lola is resting on her knuckles in the picture to ease any discomfort in the wrist. The soft ball is placed between the thighs to aid activation of the pelvic floor muscles during this exercise, and to help with any discomfort of the pubic bone. Do not squeeze the ball too tightly if your pubic bone is painful.

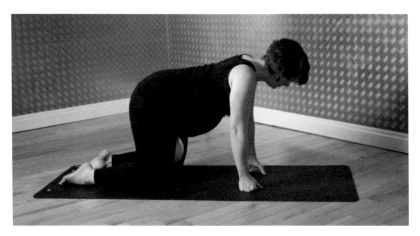

Prepare for the core cat

Prepare
Get down on your hands and knees, with your knees hip-distance apart.
Exhale as you zip up your pelvic floor by tidying up your bladder and back passage.
Keep your back and neck long.
You can place a soft ball between your thighs to help activate the inner thigh and pelvic floor muscles.
Your hands should be shoulder-distance apart, straight down from your shoulders.
Look directly at the mat.

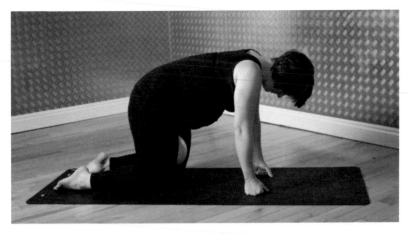

Perform the core cat

Perform the exercise
Inhale.
Exhale as you draw your tummy muscles in to hug your baby into your back, squeezing your bladder and back passage.
Stop when feel your back begin to arch into a cat position.
Inhale, relax the tummy and pelvic floor, and return to the start position.
Do not arch your back; simply try to pull your baby into your spine using muscular contraction – as though your trousers are too tight.

Repetitions
8 repetitions × 3 sets

Breathing and pace
Try to move at the pace of your breathing. It is essential to use your full exhalation through the movement.

Progression

If you would like to work a little more intensely into the core group of muscles, you can perform this exercise with your elbows resting on a gym ball – but avoid this if your blood pressure has a tendency to be high.

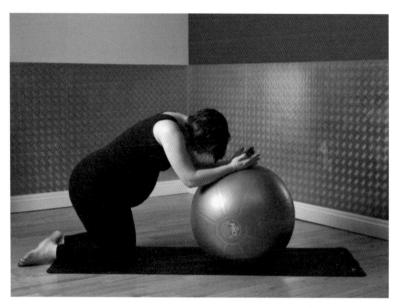

Progression of the core cat

SEATED MERMAID WAVE

This exercise, which is great for oblique and pelvic floor conditioning, can be executed in a sitting position. If your pubic bone hurts,
you can sit with straight legs. Lola has her feet together to aid engage-
ment with the pelvic floor.

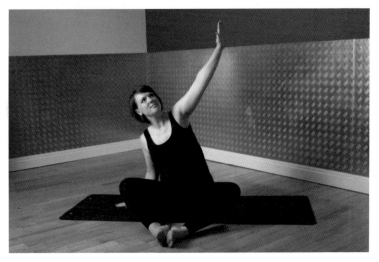

Perform the seated mermaid wave (left arm)

Prepare

Sit upright and place your feet together or sit with straight legs (place
a soft ball or cushion under your hips for support if required).
Inhale.
Exhale as you tidy up your pelvic floor.
Keep your back and neck long and tall.

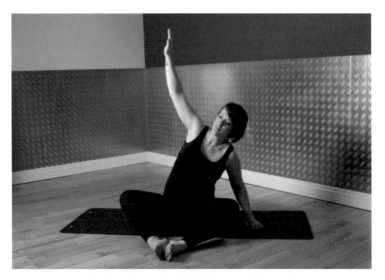

Perform the seated mermaid wave (right arm)

Perform the exercise
Inhale.
Exhale as you place one hand on the floor and reach to the ceiling
with the other.
Your challenge is to keep your pelvic floor tidy during this whole
movement.
Inhale then repeat.
Stop if feel your back begin to slouch.

Repetitions
8 repetitions × 3 sets for each arm

Breathing and pace
Try to move at the pace of your breathing. It is essential to use your
full exhalation through the movement. Each inhalation and exhalation is a movement in this exercise.

Progression

If you find this seated mermaid wave too easy, try this sideways seated version.

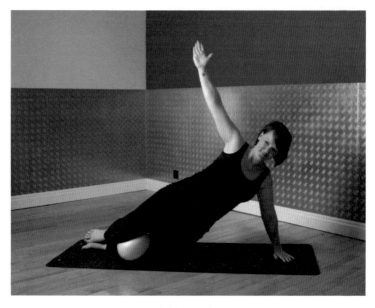

Progression of the seated mermaid wave

If you suffer from high blood pressure, please avoid this progression.

You can keep a soft ball or cushion between your knees to ensure alignment for the pelvis.

Inhale and tidy up the pelvic floor.

Exhale while elevating the hips off the floor and reaching one arm up towards the ceiling.

Inhale to return.

Repetitions

Repeat 5 times each side

SPINAL MOBILISATION AND WAIST TWIST

This exercise is good for mobilising your spine and utilising the oblique muscles of the core.

Prepare
Sit upright with legs straight out in front of you. Place a cushion under your bottom if you struggle to sit upright, and hold a soft ball between your hands to encourage you to sit tall.
Inhale.
Exhale as you tidy up your pelvic floor.
Keep your back and neck long and tall.

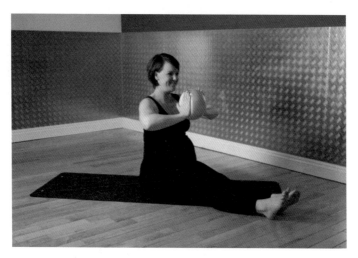

Prepare for spinal mobilisation and waist twist

Perform the exercise
Inhale.
Exhale as you elevate your elbows to shoulder height and rotate at the waist.
Keep the ball in line with the chest as you turn to the side.
Inhale to return.

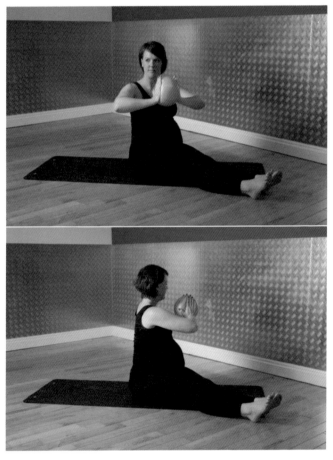

Perform spinal mobilisation and waist twist

Repetitions
Repeat 8 times each side

Breathing and pace
Try to move at the pace of your breathing. It is essential to use your full exhalation through the movement.
Your challenge is to keep your pelvic floor tidy during this whole movement.
Note: Stop if you feel your back begin to slouch.

Progression
Place the soles of your feet together to make this exercise a little more challenging.

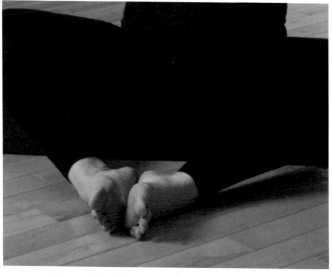

Progression of spinal mobilisation and waist twist

CHAPTER 8

Building the foundations for recovery

I have mentioned the pelvic floor often during the previous exercise pages, as it is important to engage these muscles during general exercise. It is equally important to train this muscle group in isolation, to enable you to recover after giving birth.

It is a myth that you do not need to exercise the pelvic floor if you have a caesarean section. The opposite is true. It is pregnancy that causes the initial weakness in the pelvic floor as it battles under the strain of the weight of the baby, amniotic fluid and placenta. If you fail to care for your pelvic floor, you run the risk of physiological discomfort during pregnancy, particularly in the lower back. Physiological problems after giving birth, such as bladder or bowel weakness, are also likely to occur. In extreme cases, prolapse of the bladder, bowel or uterus are a risk, all of which require surgical intervention to repair.

WHAT IS THE PELVIC FLOOR?

The pelvic floor is a group of muscles that form a sling of stability throughout the cavity of a woman's pelvis. This group of muscles is important in providing support for pelvic organs – bladder, intestines, uterus – and for continence (control of bladder and bowels). It facilitates birth by helping the foetus to rotate forwards to navigate its descent into the pelvic girdle.

The midwives of the pregnant women who have recovered well after giving birth because they have been dedicated to their fitness and pelvic health through our programme have praised our method. Pelvic floor exercises are, in my opinion, the single most important exercise *any* woman, pregnant or not, can undertake. The pelvic floor muscles are the foundations of your posture and abdominal strength. If your pelvic floor is neglected, you will only damage yourself when participating in general forms of exercise as your support structure will not be in place.

Outside of pregnancy, lower back ache can often be attributed to weakness of the pelvic floor. Women who had an epidural during labour often complain that this has given them a bad back. There can be an unusual sensation around the epidural site for a few days after labour, but back pain should not be attributed to the epidural. Muscular weakness of the abdominal core and pelvic floor is usually the culprit, coupled with poor posture during feeding and when carrying your baby in your arms.

Pelvic floor exercises are not just a short-term remedy to preparing for or recovering from delivery. The care of these muscles is a lifestyle choice. If you care for them, you are less likely to need incontinence pads in later life, or suffer surgery due to prolapse. Pelvic floor weakness can cause an inability to control flatulence too!

I teach a series of pelvic floor stability exercises based on tried and tested formulas practised by fitness and physiotherapy professionals. These are basic exercises and can be done any time of day, at any location, in any situation, with a little concentration and breathing.

POSTURE AND THE PELVIC FLOOR EXERCISES

If your posture is poor during the pelvic floor exercises, you will not effectively train your pelvic floor; you will be wasting your time and energy. It is essential to keep your spine long and tall during pelvic floor training to optimally activate these muscles. Try a test to prove this to yourself:

Stand long and tall, and squeeze your bladder and back passage muscles. Be conscious of the sensation of that contraction. Then slouch into your least elegant posture, let your tummy hang out, and round your shoulders. Now attempt to squeeze the bladder and back passage, and you will notice it is much more difficult to do so in this posture. Tip: Squeezing the bladder and back passage is the same sensation as preventing wind, the passing of a bowel movement or urine.

THE FITMAMA™ PELVIC GIRDLE STABILITY SESSION

THE TRAFFIC LIGHT TWITCH

This exercise for the pelvic floor is important to help you with problems such as leakage when sneezing, coughing, running or jumping. (If you were not already an experienced runner before pregnancy, please avoid running or jumping in pregnancy as this is dangerous for the unstable pelvis and can cause damage to the pelvic girdle.)

I call this exercise the traffic light twitch as I recommend that if you are waiting at traffic lights in your car, or waiting to walk at a pedestrian crossing, you try to see how many repetitions you can achieve in this time. If you are not likely to come across traffic lights, find other triggers to help you, such as while waiting for the kettle to boil.

Prepare

Sit comfortably. Place a cushion or soft ball under your hips behind you if it helps to sit upright.

Keep your spine long and tall.

It helps to place your hands on your baby, as you may feel the tummy responding to the pelvic floor squeezes.

The stronger the pelvic floor, the more likely you are to feel your tummy moving as you squeeze.

Perform the exercise

Intermittently squeeze your bladder and back passage muscles, then let go.

Try to squeeze a full contraction to switch on.

Try to release completely between each contraction.

If you tire, stop and try more later.

Keep breathing regularly throughout this sequence.

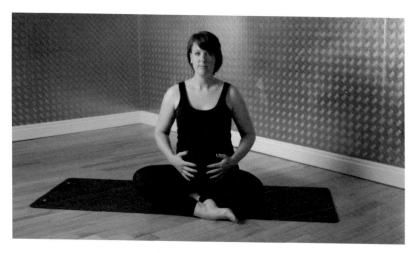

The traffic light twitch

Repetition

Ideally, try to repeat this exercise 10 times, performed 3 times per day. If you prefer, you can do this exercise in bed morning and night. If you do it lying on your side, please ensure that you turn over and repeat on the other side for good muscular balance.

THE LONG HOLD FOR ENDURANCE

This exercise for the pelvic floor is important not only to help you tone the muscle group, but to give you the advantage when you need to wait to visit the toilet. During pregnancy, the urge to get to the toilet immediately can be exacerbated by the weight of your baby and the softening of tissues in the pelvis. This exercise will help you after your baby is born too, as often the urgency to get to the toilet is increased after delivery.

You can again find a trigger to help you practise this exercise, such as squeezing your pelvic floor at traffic lights and counting to 10. See how many sets of 10 you can count during your time at the lights.

Perform the exercise
Inhale to prepare.
Exhale as you squeeze the back passage first (as though you are trying to prevent wind), then draw in the bladder muscle to create a full squeeze.
Hold for a count of 10. Use your full exhalation time to squeeze and hold.
Inhale, then exhale to completely relax these muscles.

Repetitions
Try to repeat this exercise 10 times, performed 3 times per day.
Try to combine this with the traffic light twitch for a full pelvic workout.

RELAXING YOUR PELVIC FLOOR

If you over-activate your pelvic floor by training it too hard, you can cause yourself to be mildly retentive in this area. Ideally, you want to be able to relax these muscles so that you can accommodate your baby's head and body during delivery. The pelvic floor will contract of its own accord to progress delivery of your baby.

So, once you have completed your pelvic floor exercises, take a deep breath, right into the back of your lungs, and as you exhale allow your pelvic floor to completely unwind. Try to relax the bladder and back passage completely. Imagine that your pelvic floor becomes so relaxed your baby could simply slide out with ease.

Being able to relax your pelvic floor will go a long way to helping you manage the phases of labour between contractions, and to help your baby descend into the pelvis.

Top tip
Remember, even if you become bed-bound during your pregnancy, these exercises can still be done – unless absolutely contraindicated by your physician or midwife. If you do nothing else during pregnancy, these pelvic floor exercises will create some stability in your pelvis and some muscle tone to help your baby on the journey out.

CHAPTER 9

To stretch or not to stretch?

There is plenty of debate in the world of pregnancy exercise as to whether or not stretching-style exercises are safe. Some opinions may be that yoga in pregnancy is not safe due to the extreme positions involved, in which muscles are lengthened. This could pose a painful problem, as during pregnancy the ligaments suffer from excessive levels of the hormone relaxin. Over-stretching could cause the ligaments to become unstable and create long-term, painful damage.

Another school of thought is that stretching in pregnancy is good and helps the mother to be calm and flexible.

My opinion is somewhere in the middle. I believe that stretching should be undertaken in a controlled way, emphasising maintenance and avoiding progressive stretching which could damage the ligaments. I want you to release the muscles of tension, but keep the ligaments and tendons safe.

The safest way to achieve this is to rely on how the stretching feels to you. If you are stretching your legs and the backs of your knees feel uncomfortable, you are probably taking the stretch too far. And if you are hyper-mobile (as described in chapter 2), you will need to be extra cautious about keeping stretches sedate and within the pictorial parameters shown in this chapter.

THE FITMAMA™ SAFE STRETCH SESSION

Less is definitely more in pregnancy stretching, so don't go for the burn. Instead, try to visualise long, healthy muscles with safe, stable ligaments and tendons. Be gentle with yourself: don't push or pull too hard.

Clear, fluid breathing is required during these stretches. Pelvic floor muscles should be tidied up to ensure support of the pelvic girdle during the exercises. Focus on your posture to keep the stretch safe, and listen to your body. If anything hurts, stop!

If you over-stretch during pregnancy, you will be setting yourself up for aches and pains in your postnatal time – particularly if you breastfeed, because the instability caused by relaxin will still be present in your body. By following the safe stretch, you will be saving yourself ligament and tendon trauma, which often revisits us in later life when our joints begin to play up.

CHEST STRETCH

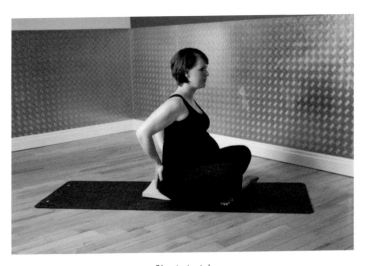

Chest stretch

Perform the exercise
Sit comfortably, with your hands placed on your lower back.
Lift your chest and feel the opening of your chest area.
Hold for about 10 to 15 seconds.

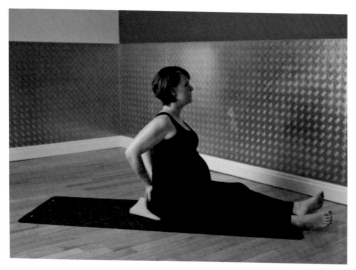

Progression of chest stretch

Progression

You can add to your chest stretch by extending your legs out in front of you. You will notice that as you sit upright, you will feel a release at the back of the thighs.

If you flex your feet and pull them towards your tummy, you will feel the release travel to your calf muscles.

Hold for about 10 to 15 seconds.

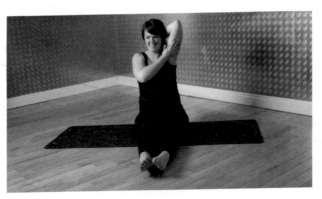

Triceps (back of arm) stretch

TRICEPS (BACK OF ARM) STRETCH

Continue to sit tall, with your legs out in front of you or crossed if you find that more comfortable.
Place one hand behind your head; press gently with the other hand on the back of the arm to release the muscles of the triceps.
Hold for about 10 to 15 seconds. Repeat using the other arm.

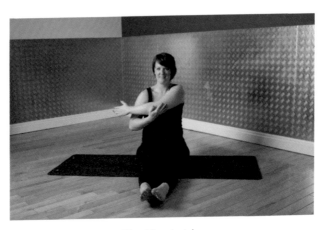

Shoulder stretch

SHOULDER STRETCH

Continue to sit tall, with your legs out in front of you or crossed if you find that more comfortable.

Take one arm across your chest; press gently with the other hand on the back of the arm to release the muscles of the shoulder.
Hold for about 10 to 15 seconds. Repeat using the other arm.

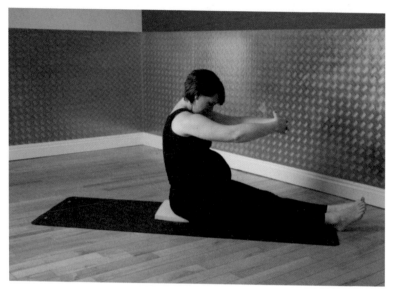

Upper back/neck stretch

UPPER BACK/NECK STRETCH

Continue to sit tall, with your legs out in front of you or crossed if you find that more comfortable.
Link your hands together in front of your chest.
Bring your chin to your chest and feel the release of your upper back and back of the neck.

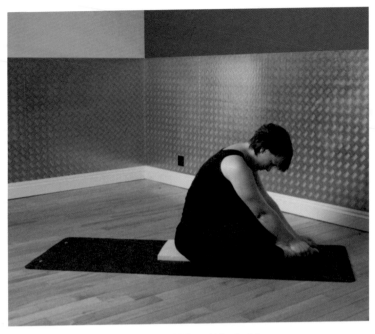

Spine, inner thigh and hip stretch

SPINE, INNER THIGH AND HIP STRETCH

If you are able sit in this position, place the soles of your feet together.

Place your hands on your feet.

Create a 'C' shape with your spine around your baby.

Feel the release through your spine, inner thighs and hip joints.

Hold for about 10 to 15 seconds each side.

Note: If you cannot put your feet together, have your legs out in front of you instead and simply place your hands on your thighs to create a 'C' shape through the spine.

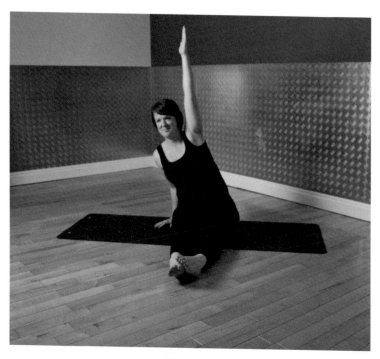

Side stretch

SIDE STRETCH

Continue to sit tall, with your legs out in front of you or crossed if you find that more comfortable.

Raise one hand directly towards the ceiling, resting the other hand on the floor.

Feel the release through the waistline.

Hold for about 10 to 15 seconds each side.

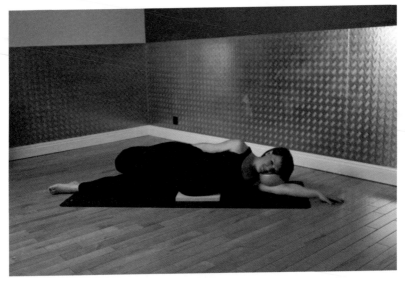

Quadriceps (front of thigh) stretch

QUADRICEPS (FRONT OF THIGH) STRETCH

Lie on one side, resting your head on a cushion or soft ball and an outstretched arm for added alignment.
Support your tummy with a cushion.
Keep your knees together as you take the top foot behind you.
If you can't reach your ankle as Lola can, you can loop your exercise band around your foot as an adaptation.
Feel the release in the front of the thigh.
Hold for about 10 to 15 seconds each side.

Your stretch session should leave you feeling calm and relaxed. You can perform these maintenance stretches daily, or as and when you feel your muscles are tight. Definitely do these after you have performed any other exercise routine in this book.

The labour techniques

CHAPTER 10

Breathe your baby out

You may have seen movie scenes of actresses simulating labour and childbirth, panting and screaming at the camera, and with one dramatic, tooth gritting push, the 'baby' is delivered onto set.

These rather dodgy imitations of what actually happens in the delivery suite are usually far from the truth. Women will push for anything up to two hours in a normal delivery situation. Some will scream, some will be silent, some will whimper, and others, like me, will 'moo' like a cow.

You may have heard of the mysterious 'urge to push'. Many women feel this urge, a sensation which can only be described as like the muscular contraction one feels when about to vomit – the difference being that the muscle contractions are working in the opposite direction. The urge to push can be completely overpowering, and some women will feel this prematurely. But the premature urge to push can be dangerous. If your midwife tells you that it is not time to push, right at the moment you have the urge, please listen and try to practice the 'push urge' control breathing mentioned in this chapter. If you push when advised not to, you could tear your cervix, or cause difficulties for your baby if the baby's shoulders are stuck. Tearing the cervix will require surgery immediately after delivery, leaving your birth partner holding the baby – worse still, dressing the baby! Who knows what outfit the baby could be presented to the world in?

Breathing will help you to control how your muscles respond to the various stages of your labour and delivery. To put it in simple terms, when you exhale, the oxygen you have breathed in is passed from the lung cavity into the bloodstream and carried directly to the muscles and organs. Imagine it is the same as driving your car: as you press your foot onto the accelerator, the fuel is taken to the engine to make it work. So, if you hold your breath you will be starving your body of its fuel. Breathing is the accelerator of delivery. You know that when you drive you are in control of how fast or how slowly your vehicle goes; the same can apply to your labour.

I apply three different styles of breathing to labour practice:

- Relaxation breathing
- 'Push urge' control breathing
- Push to deliver breathing: phase one and phase two

These styles of breathing are designed to help you through the various stages of your labour. The techniques are designed to help you cope with and manage your delivery more effectively. You will feel a sense of control if you practise these breathing techniques beforehand.

They can also be used throughout your pregnancy to help you during stressful or physically uncomfortable situations. Relaxation breathing can help you when you feel upset, scared, panicked, angry, or if you have had a sudden burst of adrenaline – which can be quite frightening. The 'push urge' control breathing can help you if you are suffering from very strong Braxton Hicks contractions (a tightening of the uterus which can feel like a real contraction, usually felt during the third trimester but which can be felt much earlier) or if you are in pain when passing bowel movements.

Speaking of bowel movements . . . there is a chance that, when you are nearing the end of your delivery time, you will feel the urge to pass a bowel movement or 'poo'. This is often quite an alarming prospect for women, as our modesty is potentially compromised – especially as in many cases our birth partner is the love of our life and we would feel mortified to poo in front of them! But please don't panic. The sensation of needing to pass a movement is very often just that, a sensation. As your baby's head descends past the bowel the nerve endings of the bowel will respond and make you feel as though you need to pass a motion. This is a point at which some women will panic and hold back. Don't! This is a sign that your baby is about to be born . . . embrace that sensation and keep going with the urge to push, or instructions to push from your midwife.

Even if there is some excrement in your back passage, the baby's head will push it out of the way in order to descend and be born. If this is the case, midwives are amazing at keeping your modesty intact: they will whisk the evidence away before anyone has had a chance to notice, not least for the health and safety of your new baby.

So remember, the urge to poo means that your baby is about to be born. If you feel it, tell your midwife . . . be brave, listen to your midwife and *breathe and push!*

THE FITMAMA™ BREATHING TECHNIQUES

We know that breathing is essential for life, but did you know that breathing can help you to manage pain and stress? As you exhale, the exchange of oxygen from the lungs into the bloodstream takes place, sending fuel to the muscles. Not only does this help you during exercise, but it can help you during painful moments of labour. Sending oxygen to the muscles during a contraction, for example, can help you to relax into the contraction.

Fighting contractions will only make them more intense and painful, so learn to breathe the pain away! Tension in the mouth creates tension in the abdominal core and the pelvic floor, so relaxing the tongue and jaw will help you to relax through the breathing techniques and processes of labour, enabling your birth canal to relax enough to accommodate your baby's descent.

Remember, the pain of contractions is a *good* sign! It indicates that your body is working hard to expel your baby from your womb, so that you can finally hold your baby in your arms. Contractions are your communication link to what is happening to your body during labour.

I often tell the women I work with to practise these techniques when on the toilet. Passing a difficult bowel movement is a perfect opportunity to practise these techniques.

It is also a good idea to learn these techniques with your birth partner, so they can remind you of how to breathe when you are overwhelmed with the job of labour.

RELAXATION BREATHING

This technique can be used during the quiet phases of your labour, to help keep your mind focused, calm and positive. Often we feel overwhelmed and afraid of the unknown during labour, but practising rhythmical calm breathing will go a long way to helping you stay rational and relaxed.

Perform the breathing

Slowly allow your inhalation to trickle in through your nose.

Visualise filling your lungs up from the very bottom of the lung cavity, widening your ribs as the lungs expand with oxygen.

Soften your jaw (don't bite your teeth together) and allow your tongue to rest relaxed in your mouth.

Allow the breath to be released through your mouth, with soft lips.

Be conscious of your facial muscles relaxing, your shoulders relaxing, and your tummy muscles softening.

Imagine that with every gentle exhalation your baby descends with ease into the pelvic cavity and slides easily into the birth canal.

Top tip: This relaxation breathing is perfect for the administration of the epidural needle. The consultant may ask you to inhale before the needle is inserted. Slowly trickle your breath out as the needle goes in between the vertebrae of your spine, helping you to relax and not make any sudden movements while this delicate procedure takes place. The sensation of the needle going in is not painful, just odd-feeling.

'PUSH URGE' CONTROL BREATHING

This technique can be used if you are experiencing an urge to push but your midwife has asked you not to push yet. Her reasons may be that your cervix is not ready or your baby may need some more time before you push.

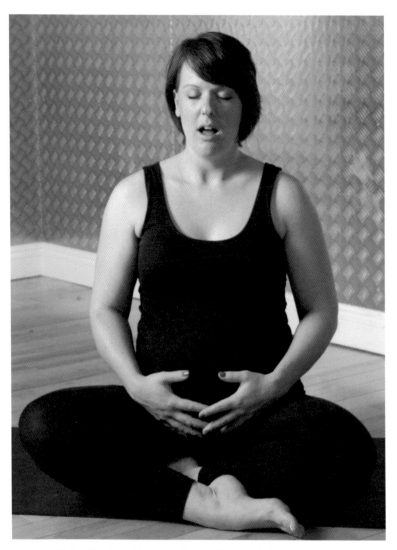

Relaxation breathing: visualise meeting your baby and breathe!

Perform the breathing

Inhale deeply through your nose.

Soften your jaw and relax your mouth into a happy face.

Pant the breath out in five sharp exhalations: 'HAH HAH HAH HAH HAH' or 'HEE HEE HEE HEE HEE'.

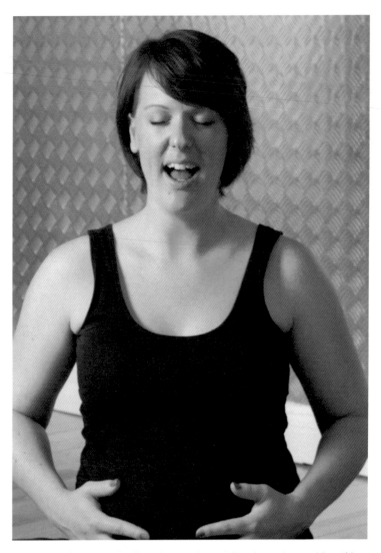

Lola relaxes her jaw and softens her mouth to aid 'push urge' control breathing.

Visualise with every pant that you are stepping away from the over-whelming contractions of your abdomen.

Visualise that every pant minimises the 'push urge' sensation and helps you to regain control.

A relaxed happy face will help to relax the pushing muscles.

The release of oxygen into your bloodstream through this breathing will help to minimise the contracting of the muscles, thereby helping the urge to push to decrease.

Top tip: This type of breathing is perfect if you experience pain when visiting the toilet. It can help the bowel muscles relax so that you can comfortably empty your bowels.

PUSH TO DELIVER BREATHING

Some women will feel that they have failed if they push for some time and then need some intervention to help the baby out. Please don't be so hard on yourself. You are doing all the right things, and sometimes, nature just plays games with us. Larger babies often need intervention if their shoulders are too broad to allow easy exit from the birth canal. Sometimes you can push for so long that exhaustion simply dictates that you need help.

There is no perfect scenario. Go with the flow, do your best, and take the help that is offered if you need it. Don't be a maternity martyr!

There are conflicting opinions about breathing techniques for pushing. Some professionals feel that if you hold your breath during the pushing process, you may cause damage to the rectus abdominis muscles (these run from the pubic bone to the sternum). In my opinion, any damage done to muscles is often down to genetics, hyper-mobility and size of uterine contents (baby, fluid, placenta). Most women will suffer more damage if they have not been active during pregnancy and have not prepared the muscles for pushing, as I teach in this book.

It is very easy to feel confused by all the opinions out there. As much as we encourage you to be upright and breathe to push your baby out, this may not be possible for you in the end, and you may need to lie on your back and use the 'breath hold' technique if directed to do so by your midwife.

Holding your breath as you bear down and push could make the difference between needing assisted delivery or not. The power behind the push is increased when the oxygen is stored in the lungs at the moment of pushing. The repair of diastasis (separated muscles) is far preferable to surgical intervention for delivery. But this is a personal choice.

A midwife I know through my work says that trying to deliver using different positions and postures is key. Sometimes, depending on the baby's size and position, the strength and frequency of contractions, the shape and type of your pelvis, and the length of the second stage of labour, lying on your back and performing 'directive' pushing with a breath hold can make the difference between normal birth and being transferred to the obstetric unit. The second stage of labour can be very tiring and sometimes women need that extra bit of encouragement.

My advice is to try everything and rule out nothing!

I have broken the push to deliver breathing technique into two phases.

PUSH TO DELIVER BREATHING: PHASE 1

This works with the flow of your natural breathing. You can use it in the early stages of teasing the baby down your birth canal using relaxed pushing, without holding your breath.

Perform the breathing
Inhale calmly through your nose.
Exhale as you shorten the space between your ribs and your hips, creating a 'C' shape with your spine, tucking your chin into your chest. Hug your bump with your body.
Blow the air out with real energy as you push your baby toward the vaginal exit by bearing down into your back passage. Let your voice be heard; it helps with your pushing to make a noise.
Your final pushes will deliver your baby into the world; you can use phase two for these.

PUSH TO DELIVER BREATHING: PHASE 2

This breathing is great for that final hurdle when you know your baby is about to emerge and you need a little extra power to push! You can hold your breath for this phase.

Be prepared to do this more than once as your baby plays the cat and mouse game, slipping back a fraction into the birth canal with each push.

Perform the breathing

Take a large gulp of breath into the lungs; open your mouth to do this.

Hold your breath as you shorten the space between your ribs and your hips, creating a 'C' shape with your spine, tucking your chin into your chest. Hug your bump with your body.

Blow the air out with real energy as you push your baby to birth by bearing down into your back passage.

You will feel a burning sensation around your vagina as the baby's head crowns and passes through the vaginal opening. This is the sensation of the skin stretching – a great sign that it's nearly over! Work with it and *push!*

Once you have delivered, be prepared to push a little more to help deliver your placenta within 15 to 20 minutes of birth.

Top tip: Pushing needs to be done as though you are pushing out a bowel movement, so when you are on the toilet is a good time to practice the push to deliver breath. Pretend your bowel movement is your practice labour. Just try not to push too hard until the actual labour day! Allow your vocal cords to work as you push, make a noise; it does help to activate the pushing mechanism and your diaphragm is then allowed to get involved with the push. The diaphragm is part of your core group of abdominal muscles.

UNEXPECTED ISSUES

If your baby is a little stuck, or has the cord around its neck, your midwife may ask you to pant again. Please listen to this instruction, as it will help you to avoid pushing at a crucial moment when your baby may need attention. Trust yourself and listen to your midwife.

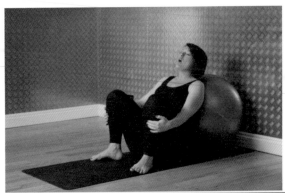

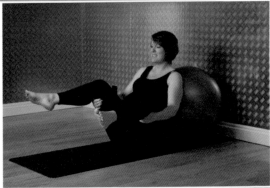

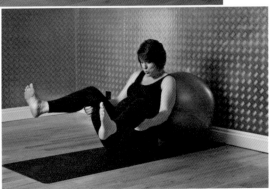

This is it! Push your baby OUT!

CHAPTER 11

Move it, baby!

If you are well during labour, and not under epidural or foetal monitoring, I advise you to try to keep mobile as much as you can. Keeping mobile will help to progress your labour and give your baby more opportunity to make an effective descent into the birth canal.

But keeping mobile should not mean exhausting yourself before your energy is required for delivery. Accordingly, I have devised some practical and easy movement techniques to help keep you mobile, progress your labour and effectively manage your labour with activity.

Please remember to rest between periods of activity. Keep hydrated, and try to snack if your energy levels are feeling depleted. Remember, hydration will help to alleviate exhaustion, so sips of water throughout labour will be useful.

THE FITMAMA™ MOVEMENT TECHNIQUES

You can choose one or a mixture of all these techniques, so practise them at home and find which ones work for you. The techniques are meant to help you remain calm, so focus on your relaxation breathing through all of these movements to help create positive, calm energy for both you and your baby.

THE BODY WRAP

Perform the movement
Stand tall.
Sway from side to side.
Wrap your arms around yourself as you shift your weight from side to side, but allow your arms to be loose, like a rag doll.
Keep both feet in contact with the floor.
The pace is steady and moves in time with your breathing:

inhale to sway one way, exhale to sway the other way.

If this movement makes you feel a little dizzy, look straight ahead and visualise your baby making the descent to birth with every sway and exhalation.
Stop when you tire and feel the need to rest.

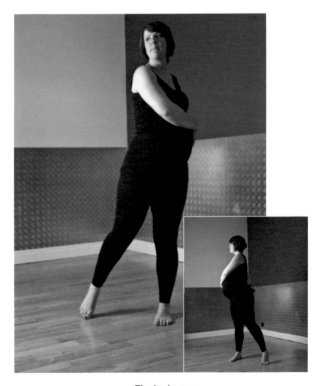

The body wrap

THE FLOATING SQUAT

Perform the movement
Stand tall, with your feet hip-distance apart.
Sit back into a squat position.
Stand upright again, floating one leg up and away from the floor.
Sit again in a squat position.
Stand upright again, floating the other leg away from the floor.
The pace is steady and moves in time with your breathing. Inhale to sway one way, exhale to sway the other way.
If the leg lift is too much for you, just focus on the squats and gently repeat this action until you are ready to rest.
Stop when you tire and feel the need to rest, or if you feel unbalanced.

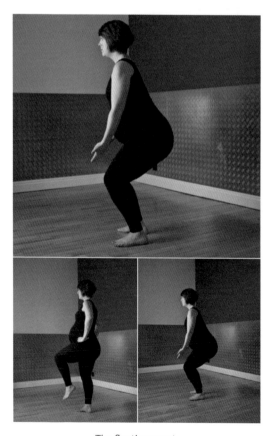

The floating squat

THE SEATED HIP SWAY

Perform the movement
Sit on a gym ball with your bare feet flat on the floor
Sit with your spine long and tall.
Inhale as you sway the hips one way.
Exhale and sway the hips the other way.

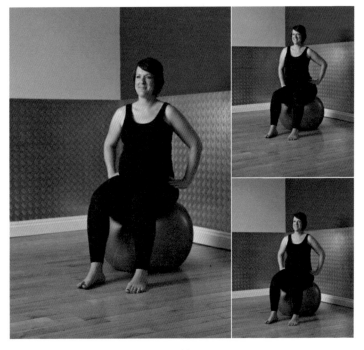

The seated hip sway

Visualise that each sway is helping your baby to creep further into the birth canal, and that every breath and sway softens and widens your pelvis in preparation for delivery.
Every breath will relax your abdominal muscles, with special focus on your pelvic floor muscles.

Progression
If you want to progress this movement, you can rock your pelvis forward and backward with each breath.

Another progression is to draw small circles with your pelvis with each breath, in each direction.

Top tip: This seated hip sway movement is very useful during pregnancy when your lower back feels uncomfortable, and can help with preparation for labour in the weeks running up to your due date.

DID YOU KNOW?

Slouching at your desk or on the sofa encourages your baby to slump into a back to back position, making delivery all the more difficult for you both. Consider sitting on a gym ball at your desk to help avoid this and tilt your pelvis into the correct position. You could even do your hip sways and pelvic floor exercises seated on the ball at work!

THE REST SWAY

If you are exhausted but want to keep moving, you can rest your chest and head against a ball, place a cushion or soft ball between your feet and bottom, and allow your body to sway gently from side to side. This will help you regain some energy, while keeping your labour active.

Top tip: This position will help to optimise the position your baby faces for delivery, and is a great position during pregnancy to find relief from back ache.

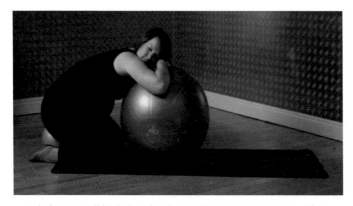

Lola has a small ball placed under her bottom to help with comfort.

CHAPTER 12

Push it real good:
choosing a delivery position

You may feel confused by the positions available for delivery. I would suggest that you don't decide on a position beforehand, but practise getting into a few different positions to familiarise yourself with the options.

There is a belief that delivering on your back is not recommended. But in both my deliveries I ended up on my back due to pure exhaustion. That's not to say that I didn't labour in plenty of other positions, from standing to kneeling and frankly, rolling around like a ball in confusion during the rather emotional stages of my labours.

The fitter and stronger you are, the more stamina you will have for the more upright positions for labour. For example, if you have exercised your legs with the routines described in chapter 5, you will find that you have more stamina to deliver your baby in a standing position, resting your back against the wall.

If you have exercised your abdominal and pelvic floor muscles as described in chapters 7 and 8, you will find you have more power in these areas and will be able to push more effectively using the positions in this chapter.

PRACTISING POSITIONS FOR DELIVERY

Get into the habit of trying out these positions, and practise them in conjunction with your breathing techniques. The more you practise, the more natural they will feel when you are in labour and ready to deliver.

THE LOLA

This position is fondly named after our lovely FitMama™ model Lola Turvey, who used this position to deliver her son Charlie.

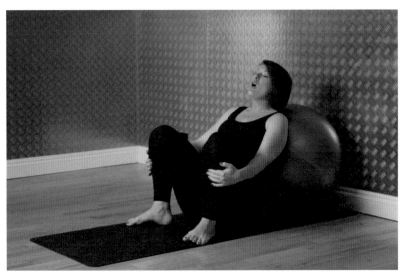

The Lola (inhalation)

Lola has drawn her knees close to her with her legs wide open.

- She takes a deep inhalation.
- She brings her chin to her chest, creating a 'C' shape around her baby.

- She exhales as she bears down to push her baby out with power, focusing on pushing into her bottom, lifting her feet and supporting her thighs with her hands.

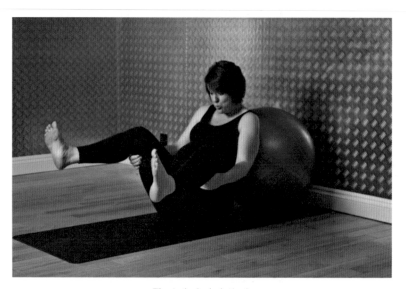

The Lola (exhalation)

THE WALLFLOWER

In an upright position, gravity plays a great role in helping your baby to make an effective descent and exit. The midwife is able to help ease your baby into the world from the birth canal.

If you have practised your leg exercises as set out in chapter 5, you will find this position much easier to endure for a longer period of time. The muscles of your legs will be better able to support the weight of you and your pregnant belly.

You could lean in an upright position with your birth partner standing behind you and supporting your body. However, he or she will be exhausted after a while, so this position against a wall leaves your birth partner and midwife free to concentrate on actively helping you deliver your child.

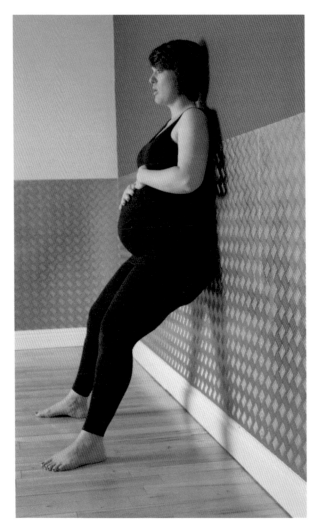

The wallflower

- Lola takes a deep inhalation.
- She brings her chin to her chest, creating a 'C' shape around her baby.
- She exhales as she bears down to push her baby out with power, focusing on pushing into her bottom.

THE DELIVERY CAT

This position can be assumed on the floor, or even on the delivery bed, using either a ball for resting support or the moveable head of the bed if in a delivery suite. 'The delivery cat' can be very helpful if you are suffering from lower back pain during labour.

- Lola takes a deep inhalation.
- She brings her chin to her chest, creating a 'C' shape around her baby.
- She exhales as she bears down to push her baby out with power, focusing on pushing into her bottom.

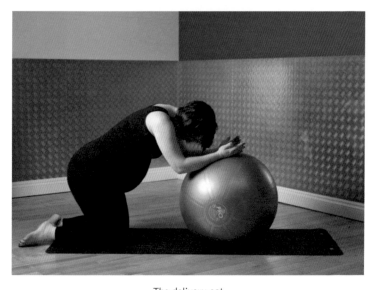

The delivery cat

THE HYPNOBIRTHER

Some women are able to deliver in a completely relaxed state, using breathing techniques and affirmations to control their delivery. The mind is an amazing tool, and if you can trust your body to know what it is doing while using your mind to repeat positive thoughts to yourself, you will find your labour a calm and manageable process.

I have worked with women who have managed to deliver their babies in a completely passive state in this recovery style position.

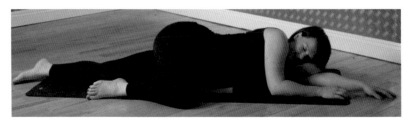

The hypnobirther

REAL MUMS' POSITIONS

Whichever position you end up in, the good news is that the end of this physical challenge is near, and your new challenge of motherhood and recovery is about to commence!

To help you get an idea of how position can impact on your labour and birth, here are some of the comments about birth positions our FitMama™ participants have shared with us via the Facebook group.

On my back first time (no choice as hooked up to all sorts) and sort of half-sitting the second. It just felt like the position I had the most control in.

Claire E

I invented 'The Lola' with my first, Charlie, and then I had no choice with Freddie, I was on my back with the midwife pumping my legs like a water pump!

Lola, FitMama™ trainer

Kneeling on hospital bed with arms dangling over the headrest.

Gillian E

At first on all fours, then on my side (with my husband next to me, holding my hand). The final stage I ended up on my back rather than in the birthing pool, as Louis decided to make a fast appearance. It was the best position for me, being able to breathe down towards the baby . . . just like Marie taught us.

Anna-Sophie S-B

First one kneeling, second one on my back due to complications and rapid delivery!

Toni B

I was on my knees but it really worked for me as I was able to push downwards. I did not feel that comfortable sitting up.

Vicki H

On my back, sitting up, as I'd been in labour so long I gave up and opted for the epidural. In all fairness I was so tired by that point I had to be manhandled across the bed to even have the epidural. Planned position was to be resting over the back of the bed, kneeling.

Natalie E

Resting over back of bed on knees for both of mine.

Gemma H

My plan was the same as Gemma's; however, I had to be on my back due to long labour and other reasons; there was no choice!

Helena V-F

Sitting on the birth stool!

Catalina S

First baby on my side gripping gas and air for dear life, and with second on my back with an epidural and my ankles pulled almost behind my ears!

Jennifer W

Squatting in the pool ... primitive!

Bronwyn M-B

CHAPTER 13

Can you handle the sharp end?

This chapter is dedicated to the special person you will take into the delivery environment with you, whether it be baby's daddy, your mum, your dad, sister or close friend.

As birth partner, you need to have the special skill of being able to dodge, or take on the chin, any insult or piece of medical equipment which may be thrown at you. This may be more of a requirement if you are the father of the baby and have not quite fulfilled the check-list of expectations during the pregnancy to date. Did you go to the 24-hour garage to purchase an ice-cream at 3 am every time the craving overwhelmed your baby's mother? If you can answer yes, you are probably safe.

Teasing aside, your expectant partner will be entering a roller-coaster ride of feelings and emotions as her labour begins and progresses. There will be moments of fear, anxiety, elation, excitement, exhaustion, panic, to name just a few. She will be feeling vulnerable, and exposed, as this is the least ladylike phase of her life, with medical staff examining her internally at every opportunity. One of my FitMama™ mums once loudly declared, 'My personal favourite was when the obstetrician donned his surgical head-lamp, slipped his hand into a surgical glove, and in front of my baby's daddy said, "Right, let's see what we have up here then!" as he went in for a full investigation of my cervix!'

Your role as birth partner is extremely important, even though you may feel like a spare wheel in the whole process – particularly if your attempts at comforting said mummy are met with snarling teeth and vile insults in one breath, then weeping and feelings of fear in the next. You are about to enter a zone which can only be understood by fellow birth partners, each with their own tale to tell.

Your patience and understanding may be put to the ultimate test. The labour could be long and exhausting for you both, and you are likely to be extremely bored during the wait. But if you are bored, you may be in danger of causing the labouring mum some distress if you decide to disappear from the delivery suite to entertain yourself. Try to use this 'boring' time to reminisce together and talk about your plans for the baby, or even have a bit of a gossip about friends and family.

Your greatest role during the active stages of delivery is to help with basic tasks:

* I advise you to practise the *breathing techniques* from chapter 10 together during pregnancy as you may need to remind the labouring mum how to breathe and when. (You can practise these yourself while on the toilet passing a bowel movement. This will help you to have some understanding of how the breathing works.)
* While she has the energy, help to keep her mobile. Gentle movement as outlined in chapter 11 is suitable, as is simply walking the corridors together. Stay with her at all times when walking.
* Keep the gas and air mouthpiece available so you can pass it to the labouring mum.
* Be close at hand to reassure her, pass anything to her, or help the midwife with anything she may need you to assist with.
* Remain calm, and talk in gentle tones so as not to distress the labouring mum. They can feel extremely sensitive. Tones like those you'd use when egging on your football team may not go down well during labour – and I speak from experience!
* You may need to speak for your labouring mum if she is in distress. Make sure you have a full understanding of what she wants before you do.
* Some mums may like to have some comforting massage during labour; others will want to hit you over the head with

the gas and air canister if you touch them. It's a risk you take, as most women won't know if they want to be touched until the moment you lay hands on them. It's not you, it's the labour!

- If there is a written birth plan, the labouring mum absolutely has the right to completely change her mind. So if she's screaming for an epidural and this is not in the plan, don't say, 'But darling, what about the birth plan?' Instead, try to discuss the issue and establish if she has truly changed her mind.
- Trust the midwifery team; they do have your labouring mum's best interests at heart. But if the ward is very busy, you may find that you need to speak up if she is in distress and there is no immediate assistance.
- To cut the umbilical cord or not? This is a personal choice, but no one will hold it against you if you prefer not to. The same applies to staying up at the head end of the labouring mother. Not all birth partners want to see the baby's head crowning. It's your choice.
- After birth, you may be left holding the baby if the baby's mum needs to have any medical attention. Don't be afraid. Keep calm, and if you feel worried ask for some help from staff on the delivery ward.

TIPS FOR BIRTH PARTNERS FROM FORMER FITMAMAS™

The following are some of the tips for birth partners left on our Facebook Group by former FitMama™ participants:

Birth partners need to be calm, supportive, positive, flexible and collected. They also need to be able to mind-read exactly what the mum to be wants/doesn't want!

Jennifer W

Remind your partner to breathe. I kept forgetting in the middle of contractions! Also, ensure they stay hydrated by giving them water through a sports bottle or straw.

Natalie E

Be flexible. Massage hard, not soft! Believe in your partner, listen to her, reassure her, touch her, arrange pillows, offer ice chips, help with position changes, be led by the midwife, never assume she will not change her mind, talk softly, be positive. There are *no failures in childbirth!*

Emma Thorpe, midwife and mum

I'm currently in hospital being induced and would say all partners should avoid sarcasm at all costs! He thinks it's helpful but it's not! Early days at the moment so she will hopefully arrive tomorrow.

Liz B

(Liz eventually gave birth after many Facebook updates.)

My birth partner said the main thing for him was the food. Cereal bars, crisps and easy snacks were not enough. He wishes he had taken advantage of the microwave available. He didn't want to leave my side so the restaurant wasn't an option for him. He thinks if he had been better fed, he wouldn't have been as tired as he would have had the energy to cope. I remember how much I appreciated having him there all the time and making me laugh. We brought music and danced as much as we could. We even used the sick bowls as party hats! A good laugh will help a lot!

Sabrina G

My husband counted for me when I got to the pushing stage, and it really helped me push for longer and see a break coming soon.

Alexandra R

Tell your birth partner who you want them to be with if mum and baby need to be separated.

Wendy D

In the last stages they need to be at your ear repeating everything the midwives are telling you to do. His was the only voice I could hear and it kept me calm and focused.

Rachel K

Tell them not to ask 'Does it hurt?'

Marie M

Take a list of family numbers so birth partner can let people know when baby born. Keep them posted if in a long labour too!

Vicky H

Make sure they have their own hospital bag (snacks, change of clothes, food – as you will be fed and they will not). Make sure they also have, understand and are in charge of the birth plan.

Gill E

Remember labour at the very worst is only one minute contraction, one minute rest, so don't be afraid. Husbands, count out the seconds for her, so that she knows it is coming to an end. Take food/drinks to the hospital; keep hydrated, you are going to be tired by the end of it. Wear comfortable cotton clothing; maternity sections in hospitals are ridiculously warm.

Ladies, despite what people say, it is possible to have a baby and not lose your dignity – wear loose clothing and speak up if you feel uncomfortable.

Vicky A

Adam was in charge of the TENS machine. I told him when a contraction was coming and he would 'burst' it for me. Also, partners need to hold your hand and cope with long, strong squeezes. He also reminded me of breathing. We practised at home – however, four days of contractions gave us lots of opportunities for practice!

Helena V-F

We found having face-to-face contact helped so that my husband could read my facial expressions. Make sure the gas and air doesn't run out, and help with the breathing. Basically, be there and have everything you might want to hand: water, music, food etc.

Katy H

Your birth partner needs to be your voice – to know when to ask the medical staff questions or chase them up. Also, it's worth getting them to watch a couple of birth/baby programmes so they know what's ahead.

Kate S

My delivery was so quick there wasn't really a chance for my husband to do anything – so my advice to all birth partners would be to go with the flow of what is happening on the day, listen to the midwives and above all, stay calm. Oh, and don't forget the camera! Ours was still in the car – lucky that phones have cameras as standard nowadays.

Georgina W

My cat's vet (don't ask how we got on to this topic with him!) gave my husband two pearls of wisdom: 1. Make sandwiches in advance and freeze them ready for the big day, because no one cares about the dad when the mum is in labour; 2. If the baby is born close to midnight, make sure you are very clear with people what the birth date is – apparently his in-laws spent the first four years of their first-born grandchild's life thinking his birthday was the day after the real day.

My personal advice would be that partners shouldn't be scared of going down the business end! I was adamant that there were some things he just shouldn't see, but actually he was really humbled by the experience of watching his child coming into the world, and I'll be more than happy for him to be down there again when number 2 arrives.

Vicki P

Huge thanks to our FitMama™ Facebook Group members for their contributions. Testament to the fact that advice from other parents is invaluable!

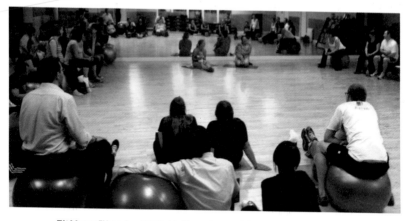

FitMama™ spring 2011 birth partners night: birthing experiences shared with our first-time parents.

CHAPTER 14

Yes, your baby needs you to relax

Pregnancy and the prospect of motherhood can be a daunting and overwhelming time for many women. Some women fly through pregnancy without a care in the world, while others will fret and worry from the very outset. This can be made worse for women who have perhaps suffered previous miscarriage or loss of a baby at any stage.

I believe the levels of stress you carry in your pregnancy will play a part in the comfort of your baby. I know this all too well from my own experiences. With my first baby, I fell into the category of mum without a care in the world. I found the pregnancy easy, hardly noticed much of a change, wore my normal clothes until seven months pregnant, and was completely naïve about the reality of labour and birth. In fact, my naïvety was perfect for the calm environment the baby needed. My baby squirmed calmly inside me and all was placid during those nine months.

My second pregnancy was a completely different story. First of all, I knew exactly what I was getting myself into. I think pregnancy the second time around is a bit alarming for women because we know what is likely to be a challenge to us in labour, so the whole pregnancy can be spent worrying about the big day. Also, my life was in a different place, with stressful changes and upheavals. My baby kicked me vigorously and let me know that she was not impressed with my distress, let alone my emotional outbursts at everything that upset me. I am sure that this is why she is so different from her brother. He was always a placid, easy to distract child. She has been intense and easy to upset from the moment she was born, bless her stomping little feet!

In this fast-paced modern world, many of us work right up to our due date. If not working, you may be at home with other children, in which case, there is no time to be pregnant. The luxury of the first successful pregnancy, where you can go to bed at 7 pm if you desire, and snooze in the afternoon at weekends, is a once in a lifetime treat! Unless you are living with a god-like creature, who takes the children off your hands and brings you tea in bed . . . sigh.

I strongly believe that we do not take enough time to help ourselves unwind. So how can you ensure your pregnancy stress levels do not affect you and your baby so much? Simply by seeking opportunities to actively participate in relaxation.

This can be at bath-time, or when you climb into bed at night, or a stolen five minutes when everyone is out of the house, or even in your car during your lunch break.

Just five minutes each day will go a long way to helping to balance your stress levels and create positivity in your pregnancy, particularly if you are suffering from pregnancy-related discomfort of the pelvis and joints. These painful afflictions can be distressing in themselves.

If you find it hard to make relaxation time, I recommend you book yourself some weekly sessions with a maternity reflexologist (please ensure they are maternity qualified), as this is an intense relaxation opportunity and you will be walking on air by the time you finish. Not only that, but maternity reflexologists are thought to be able to help with other pregnancy ailments and afflictions such as pelvic pain, late babies, babies in the wrong position for delivery, etc.

I encourage you to use the process of affirmation during your relaxation. And if it helps you, play some music which will help you to clear your mind and promote feelings of calmness.

FINDING A RELAXATION NEST

The best form of relaxation will take place in a cosy, comforting place I refer to as your relaxation nest. This can be anywhere that you feel a sense of peace and comfort. My favourite relaxation nest is actually my armchair. I like to curl up in it like a cat and let myself completely drift away against the soft, well-worn cushioning. If your relaxation nest has to be inside your car, keep some pillows in the car so you can cosy yourself up and really get comfortable.

There is nothing worse than actively seeking relaxation, only to be persistently interrupted by outside distractions. To minimise this, make sure you have turned your phone to silent, closed doors and windows if you need to, and found the right volume for your music to be played. Too loud or too quiet will not help you to find your relaxation zone.

Ensure that the room temperature is just right; usually around 21°C (70°F) is a comfortable temperature to allow the body to relax. Wear clothes which will help you maintain your body temperature so that you don't get chilly as your body activity slows down.

Make sure you are hydrated before you start. Don't drink so much water that you will need to interrupt your session to visit the toilet, but drink enough so you don't feel thirsty during the session.

If there are other people in the house, let them know you are going to have your relaxation session so that they can make sure not to interrupt you.

If you are pregnant during a heatwave, you may not need a cosy place to relax but rather a cooler environment with a gentle fan to help keep your body temperature down. See how Lola has placed herself in the recovery position on her left-hand side to help her unwind in the heat of the summer photo shoot! Notice how she is supported with cushioning under her head and tummy for added comfort.

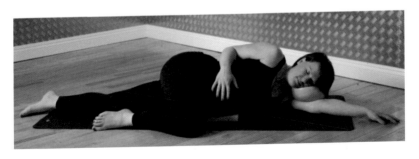

You can use this opportunity to place your hand on your tummy and create a connection between you and your baby.

THE FITMAMA™ DE-STRESS BREATHING SEQUENCE

- Slowly allow your inhalation to trickle in through your nose.
- Visualise filling your lungs up from the very bottom of the lung cavity, widening your ribs as your lungs expand with oxygen.
- Soften your jaw and allow your tongue to rest relaxed in your mouth.
- Allow the breath to be calmly released through your nose or mouth.
- Be conscious of your facial muscles relaxing, your shoulders relaxing, your tummy muscles softening, your legs becoming heavier.
- If you are lying on your left-hand side, visualise your tummy muscles softening so much that your baby slides down onto the bed or floor beside you (try not to lie on your right side as this restricts the flow of circulation).
- Allow your breathing to ebb and flow like slow gentle waves lapping at the shore.

When you're feeling comfortable in this position you can begin to mentally recite some affirmations to create a positive strength within your pregnancy, to help allay any fears or concerns you may have about becoming a mother.

THE RELAXATION AFFIRMATIONS FOR PREGNANCY

Repeat some or all of this to yourself, in any order you prefer, and feel free to alter the context of the affirmations to suit your life, or even come up with some of your own.

- I am a strong and capable woman.
- My body is healthy and well, and I nourish myself with care.
- My baby is healthy and well, and I nourish my baby with my body.
- My body knows how to carry my baby.
- My body knows how to nourish my baby.
- My baby knows how to be born.
- My body knows how to give birth to my baby.

- I trust my body to create this life, and bring my baby into this world safely.
- I trust my natural maternal instincts will come to me with ease when my baby is born.
- I trust the path I am on, and welcome my baby into my life with love and calm energy.
- I trust my midwife to guide me gently through the process of my labour.
- I trust my baby to respond to the contractions and descend into birth.
- I trust my contractions to gently expel my baby from my womb.
- I trust my body to understand the sensations of labour.
- I trust myself to be calm during labour and use the skills I have learned to cope.
- I am a strong and capable mother, who has the right to bear life and bring my baby safely into this world.
- My baby is strong.
- My body is strong.
- My womb is a safe haven for my baby until it is time for birth.
- My breathing gives life to my baby.
- My blood gives nourishment to my baby.
- My placenta supports my baby.
- My amniotic fluid cushions my baby.
- My heartbeat comforts my baby.
- I am at peace with my pregnancy.
- I love my baby.
- My baby feels my love.
- My baby feels my positive energy.
- My baby thrives when I am calm.
- I love my pregnancy.
- I love my body and trust that it will evolve as it is meant to.
- I love myself.

MEDITATION FOR PREGNANCY

You can use this meditation during pregnancy and to help you find comfort during your labour. Consider recording your own voice, to help with self-affirmation and self-comfort. You may have personal messages to yourself which you can play back to support you when you are at your most vulnerable. The reassurance of our own voice can create miracles in moments of personal challenge, like labour and delivery. If you prefer, you can ask someone you are close to if they would read the meditation for pregnancy to you.

This meditation takes you on a journey into relaxation, and the comforting low tones of a familiar voice can be extremely calming and relaxing.

Some people are not naturally inclined towards meditation, so this can be a bit of a learning curve for those of you who struggle to relax. I hope you will try to train your brain to unwind and connect to your inner consciousness. It is so good for both you and your baby to find this time. Your baby will love it, and your confidence in yourself will increase.

Go on, give it a try, and find your own way to unwind with these words.

Use your 'relaxation nest' – the cosy place you love to curl up in, or somewhere cool and quiet to help you zone out if you are pregnant in the hot months – to meditate in.

THE MEDITATION

- Now that you have found your meditation nest and are comfortable in your position, I want you to close your eyes, and be aware of the darkness behind your eyelids.
- Allow your breath to trickle slowly in through your nose, and as you exhale try to breathe out more air than you took in.
- Feel the difference between tension and relaxation now. Bite down hard on your teeth, then relax the bite. Bite down hard again, and then relax fully. Be aware of how relaxed your jaw feels when you do not bite down.
- Your jaw feels soft and supple, and this sensation begins to travel across your body with every slow breath in, and every long, calm breath out.
- As this soft, supple feeling travels through your neck and shoulder girdle, your arms become heavy, and the sockets of your shoulders are warm and relaxed.
- The soft, supple sensation creeps across your pregnant tummy, allowing your muscles to relax, thread by thread, gently

releasing your baby into a soft and supple position, both of
you feeling calm and warm.

- Your pelvis is soft and glows with warmth, your legs are heavy
  and relaxed.
- With each exhalation your body feels warm and numb, and
  the feelings of peace are deep within you and your baby.
- Your baby is responding to your state of calm with a relaxed
  face, relaxed fingers, and relaxed toes.
- Your own face, fingers and toes are warm and numb, and you
  feel completely removed from distraction around you.
- As you sink deeper into this meditation, you are one being with
  your baby. Your souls are connected and your blood pulses gently
  through your baby, giving life, nourishment, love and calm.

Be present in this moment . . . feel the life and soul you are creating,
with your own being. Feel the warmth and love, feel the uncondi-
tional bond between you and your baby, feel the peace, feel the calm,
feel the now . . .

QUICK REFERENCE CHART OF BREATHING TECHNIQUES FOR DELIVERY

Learn these breathing techniques together with your birth partner.

EARLY STAGES OF LABOUR

This technique can also be used during any time of stress during pregnancy.

Keep your jaw loose to allow the tension of your body to reduce and allow your cervix to dilate when in labour. Try to keep calm and focus on the positive meaning behind the onset of labour. Now is the time to calmly prepare your belongings for the impending birth and to keep yourself moving about to encourage the labour to progress.

- Take a long breath in through your nose.
- Loosen your jaw and exhale through your mouth.
- Keep your pelvic floor and abdominal muscles relaxed.
- Keep mobile.

'PUSH URGE' CONTROL BREATHING

You may have a premature urge to push or bear down. This sensation has a similar feeling of contraction of the abdominal muscles to when you have the urge to be sick or to pass a bowel movement. If you feel this urge and your midwife advises you it is too soon, it is essential to use the following breathing technique to avoid tearing of the cervix (this tear will result in general anaesthetic after delivery to repair the tear).

- Breathe in through your nose.
- Exhale in a panting style.
- Maintain a loose jaw and try to separate your mind from the urge.

PUSH TIME BREATHING

It is essential to use your abdominal muscles to help you push your baby out. Whichever delivery position you choose, you should be able to use this abdominal curl technique with the powerful breath of push time breathing. When pushing, try to push as though you are passing a bowel movement rather than pushing into the vagina. When you feel as though you are going to pass a bowel movement, this is usually a sign that your baby is about to be born as its head brushes past the nerves of the bowel area. Go with it and *push!*

Early pushing (phase 1)
- Breathe in deeply through your nose.
- Exhale as you tuck your chin into your chest and bear down.

Final pushes (phase 2)
- Inhale deeply through your mouth.
- Tuck your chin into your chest as you hold your breath and bear down.
- When you're ready, exhale with power, looking in the direction of the birth canal.
- Allow your body to work with the push urge.

You may feel a stinging or burning sensation around the vaginal opening as you enter the final stages of delivery. This is the sensation of the skin being stretched as your baby passes out of the birth canal. This is a wonderful, positive sign that you are about the hold your precious newborn baby! *PUSH!*

CHAPTER 15

FitMamas™ unite!

I thought you would like to read some stories from real-life FitMama™ participants to understand how the FitMama™ method of exercise and education has helped them cope with their pregnancies and early motherhood. Also, it will be interesting for you to read just how different every woman's story is.

JULIE FARRELL

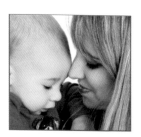

Girls, does any of this sound familiar?

In your life before bump and baby, you had a gym membership on a direct debit that you never used. You have an expensive pair of trainers for said gym membership that still look new. You own a lovely co-ordinated gym outfit. You have a sedentary office job.

All of this was me. I had a very textbook pregnancy but was plagued until 5 months with morning sickness and had a craving for anything sweet I could lay my mits on. I needed to exercise.

I bumped into an old friend by chance who recommended FitMama™, having attended classes during her own pregnancy. She said how great it had been! So I joined the antenatal class at week 30 of my pregnancy. I didn't attend any antenatal education classes via other organisations, so FitMama™ was a way for me to meet other mums as well as exercise. It got me exercising again at a late stage in my pregnancy and taught me what to actually do with the big plastic balls you see at gyms. I learnt breathing exercises, as well as hearing a variety of guest speakers on baby-related topics. The exercises gave me a taste of lots of different types of exercise such as low impact dance, yoga, tai chi, Pilates and relaxation.

I can't tell you that I magically got the exercise bug, but I understood it was essential for the wellbeing of me and my baby. I do remember one night getting ready for my weekly class. I was exhausted after a day at work. It was winter. I remember crying (thanks to hormones) whilst struggling to shave my legs over my ginormous bump, and I just wanted to curl up under the duvet . . . but I still made myself go to class!

Thanks to the skills I learnt at FitMama™, I managed to get my waters to break by using exercises on the big ball. The day before my due date I had a go on the ball and went to bed but woke up two hours later as my waters had broken. As my baby had a poo inside me I was induced using a hormone drip to speed things up. When my contractions started to hurt, I started to use the first of the breathing exercises and they really did work – so simple but effective, along with my TENS machine. It helped me to keep it together and I still felt in control. When the contractions notched up I went on to the next step of breathing and then started using gas and air. In fact, I was fully dilated using gas and air and the breathing had helped me do it as I was calm. I never in a million years would have thought I could do that, I've always had a bit of hang-up about giving birth and the pain involved.

When it was pushing time I used the last of the breathing exercises I had learnt and practised in class, but unfortunately after two hours of pushing my baby was never going to come out as he was stuck. They couldn't turn him so I had an emergency caesarean section. This was a total shock, and not something I had banked on happening to us, but it was essential for the safe arrival of my beautiful baby boy, Harry. He was a pelvic-floor-shuddering 9lb 8oz and it was love at first sight.

The caesarean knocked the stuffing out of me, and it took me a while to recover from it even with huge support from my husband and family. I still had lots of aches and pains around where I had had my surgery, and when Harry was two months old we joined FitMama™ for a postnatal course. I was really apprehensive about exercise as I was nervous about damaging my scar. Marie said she would tailor my exercises to suit as well as being able to join in with the rest of the class.

Exercise for me was the best thing for my recovery. I felt better after one week, and as I went through the course I felt better and better each time, strengthening my pelvic floor. I thought only natural childbirth affected your pelvic floor but carrying Harry for nine months and some heavy-duty pushing in labour had taken its toll. I progressed on to level two postnatal Pilates. I do still occasionally get a twinge in my scar area, but I'm six months postnatal now and through education and exercise I am managing and this is not a problem for me.

My caesarean scar has a curve to it and when I see it in the mirror it looks like a smile . . . and that smile for me really represents my whole experience of becoming a mum to Harry. Without the education I received I would have had a very different experience, and really not for the better. Thank you, FitMama™!

WENDY DALY

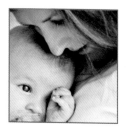

At my best before pregnancy I did two Irish dance classes a week, two combat classes and a balance class. Unfortunately, when I fell pregnant this went down to aerobics two to three times a month. Therefore I knew I would need to do something to look after myself whilst pregnant. My approach to pregnancy and labour was that you wouldn't run a marathon without training so you really shouldn't try labour without at least a few warm-up sessions.

If you have done exercise in the past you may think you don't need any specialist advice, but in pregnancy the rules change. It's not all about pushing everything to the limit. FitMama™ helped me understand my new limits, showing me how much I could do whilst pregnant but also showing me what not to do and when to stop. It helped me to familiarise myself with my changing body, and the education side of the classes helped me realise when things were wrong. I started experiencing back pain from about 20 weeks that required physiotherapy. If I hadn't attended these classes and been able to discuss this issue I probably would never have had it treated.

During my labour I experienced some difficulties. The midwife needed me to try every birthing position, to see if any of these eased the situation, before she could discuss with others what options to follow. Working on these each week in class, and my partner learning them too, on dads' night, made this a much easier and quicker process at a difficult time.

FitMama™ pelvic floor and core repair class has helped me understand the rate at which things should be repairing, and has also helped me to understand that doing too much too soon can cause problems later in life. The classes have given me confidence that things will, slowly, get back to normal.

KAREN MIDDLETON

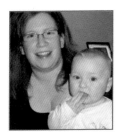

After I spent four weeks in hospital with severe oedema and high blood pressure, walking with a Zimmer frame and unable to shower or dress myself unaided, our baby girl was born. She was delivered by emergency caesarean section after a failed induction over four days. The c-section was more complicated than normal owing to the huge amount of fluid that my body was carrying, and I lost 1800 ml of blood, although they decided not to give me a blood transfusion. This was followed by a wound infection requiring IV antibiotics. I then had pancreatitis, was severely jaundiced and had pneumonia. At 10 weeks postnatal I had my gall bladder removed. At 13 weeks postnatal I joined an early postnatal pelvic floor and core repair course.

I had more to repair than the other ladies, although all of us obviously had varying levels of trauma to our bodies. By this point I was walking confidently without a Zimmer frame or walking stick, but my joints were stiff and I was wary of my balance.

The early exercises focused on pelvic floor repair and strengthening your abdominal core. This was something I felt I really needed, and I coped well with most of the exercises, with Marie tailoring exercises to my needs and ability level where appropriate. It was lovely to get to know a group of mums and for our babies to enjoy being with us. I really do feel that there is a lot of pressure for mums to join groups that stimulate babies from an early age, whereas in my opinion I think the focus should be on helping newly postnatal women to regain control of their bodies, which in turn raises confidence at a challenging time of life. The babies in our group enjoyed the interaction with other adults and babies at the beginning and end of our classes, and at any point in the class where they needed some attention – everyone benefits.

I could see an improvement in my ability every week. We all encouraged and congratulated each other at reaching our small (and big) milestones. I gradually felt more in control of my movements, and felt able to start to push myself further, although one week I was so tired I got stuck on the floor mid-exercise – Marie helped me back up and we all had a laugh, and I had a few tears of embarrassment and frustration as well. The nurturing environment of our class helped to overcome these situations, which became fewer as the course progressed.

I learnt a lot about my newly postnatal body through our instructor, and about things I should be careful of in this period of my life. I didn't realise how important pelvic floor strengthening would be to me considering I had a caesarean. I had no idea what would be appropriate exercise to begin with after my unusual ante, labour and postnatal experience. FitMama™ classes have guided me in the right direction and have encouraged me to keep working towards regaining my pre-baby level of fitness in a safe and healthy way. I am proud of the recovery I have made so far, and FitMama™ has been an important element of this.

LOLA TURVEY, FITMAMA™ TRAINER

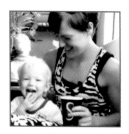

FitMama™ changed my life and made me take a completely different path to the life I had planned out.

I fell pregnant in December 2007 and was really scared about the whole prospect of leaving my career and, so I thought, my friends. I was the only one of my friends who was pregnant and none had children. I was really worried about being on my own.

FitMama™ was recommended to me by my beauty therapist, Debbie, who thought it would be good for me to meet other mothers. I was completely nervous. I had never taken part in an exercise class and I thought that I would not suit the women in the class. I was not the typical 'mummy'. However, along I went ... to the beginning of the rest of my life!

The classes were not full of what I thought was the typical mummy, but nervous pregnant women, just like me! Marie was full of confidence and was so welcoming to all of us; she really made me feel at ease. I met some wonderful people at this class and looked forward to the Tuesday night every week. The classes made me feel normal! I was a normal woman, going through pregnancy. I wasn't the only person in the world going through this! The classes taught me how to look after my growing body and how to stay healthy. I naturally became more inquisitive about the miracle of being a childbearing woman.

I had my baby and I had the usual maternity leave and went back to the usual mundane recruitment job. I got up, took my baby to nursery, came home, put baby to bed, cooked dinner, did the housework and went to bed. All of a sudden my wonderful career was just a job and the passion had gone.

I found myself thinking about FitMama™ and how the classes had really helped me mentally and physically through such an amazing time in my life. I wanted to play this part in other women's lives. I wanted to educate and help women have such an amazing journey too ... I believed this was my newfound passion.

I contacted Marie and spoke to her about how I could get involved with FitMama™. I thought I had taken her by surprise, but she said she always knew I'd be a FitMama™ trainer one day.

I studied to change my career, becoming a fitness instructor. It was worth it! I am now a pre/postnatal personal trainer and teach spin, body pump™ and body balance™ classes, and play a major part in FitMama™ antenatal and postnatal classes.

I get to bring up my two wonderful boys, Charlie and Freddie, and still hold a career doing something I truly adore. I am proud to have an impact on women's lives through the sessions in which I educate and advise them on this incredible, important time of their lives. I could not think of a job any more rewarding.

THE IMPACT OF FITMAMA™ CLASSES

I asked FitMama™ Facebook participants about how exercising during or after pregnancy, using the FitMama™ method, impacted on their lives, from all aspects. I love the fact that some of these women have not only benefited from the exercise and birthing techniques, but have in many cases made some valuable friendships to help them through the tough times of motherhood. Having someone to talk to who can relate to what you are going through will really help you to evade pre- and postnatal depression. I urge you to find some kind of class aimed at pregnant women near you, to help you with the social elements which can positively impact on your pregnancy.

Attending classes was the biggest influence for starting to get ownership of my body back.

Karen M

Getting in tune with your body before the impending birth, and of course a welcome break from the chaos at home!

Amy P

To be with other ladies in the same position as myself and having a common ground.

Laura W

In the early stages, for an hour a week I felt pregnant and normal. After three years of various fertility treatments we finally got lucky. But with my past history I decided to play my cards close to my chest, and until 20-plus weeks only a few close friends, and all the lovely FitMama™ ladies, knew. The time before the class started was great to natter to other ladies and share weekly updates. It was my only outing at that time. Marie has a lovely phrase, asking us to tuck our babies in rather than tuck in those tummies. Just that one line of hers made me believe it was all real and I was a mummy-to-be.

Kirstie S

All through pregnancy – through the stress of work and the worry of 'was everything going to be ok?' – I looked forward to the FitMama™ classes like nothing else. I met some great friends and felt like I was doing something really positive for my baby. The breathing exercises came in useful in labour – especially as it was quick and I had no time for pain relief! Really looking forward to starting postnatal classes soon.

Georgina W

I feel part of a community where everybody understands what you are going through in real time. No judgement, only understanding. I have valued learning all the breathing techniques necessary to cope during labour. I had the chance to make new friends; I am sure some will remain my friends for a lifetime. The experience is absolutely incredible and totally recommended!

Sabrina G

FitMama™ classes gave me energy and made me feel so good about myself, even though I was carrying loads of fluid. I met my best friend in the class and she has been an endless support to me over the past four years. Marie's breathing exercises got me through 20-plus hours just on gas and air, and my proudest moment was attending the class on my due date and having the energy to participate.

Anne G

FitMama™ classes introduced me to some wonderful people, two of whom I now value as close friends and see every week! My favourite parts of the sessions were the brilliant music (whenever I hear it on the radio I can't help but smile and dance!) and the warm-down where I would lie there and relax and just be at one with my baby.

Elsie B

When I was a postnatal FitMama™, my husband started to comment on my shape returning to normal after just one term of classes. I also got my core strength back and was able to play hockey after injuring myself from playing far too soon after a caesarean section. The relaxed atmosphere and the ability to feed my baby in a supportive non-judgemental environment helped increase my confidence with breastfeeding in public and showed that I could still do some exercise with my baby at my side. Mainly it was lots of fun. If you really want to know how you're progressing, then, as Marie says, just ask your husband 'Can you feel that darling?' If he says 'Feel what?' you know you still have work to do! Of course, only when you're ready!

Charlotte B

I was the first in my group of friends to fall pregnant and although it was planned, I spent the first 30 weeks or so of my pregnancy feeling slightly panicked about having a baby and cut off from my friends who didn't seem to be in a hurry to catch up. That said, I signed up to FitMama™ at about 16 weeks and really appreciated spending that hour a week with people going through the same thing as me (even if I was somewhat in awe of the calm and serene 36-plus weeks mums-to-be who turned up each week looking forward to having their babies when I definitely was not!). I met some really wonderful people and keep in touch with many of them now, even three years later.

Vicki P

I am delighted to work so closely with women who are happy to share their stories with us, and give thanks every day that I had the courage to do what I do when so many people thought I was a bit mad. It works, I love it, and I love how it can change women's lives. Thank you for taking the first step towards living a healthy motherhood. Your children will thank you for it too.

A MIDWIFE'S PERSPECTIVE

Labour is not called labour for nothing! It is a process whereby a woman's body performs its own miracle . . . a marathon which brings new life into the world – not to be underestimated. In 16 years of midwifery experience I have cared for many women who have attended pregnancy exercise programmes run by an appropriately trained instructor. One of the many things of note is that they tend to be more ambulatory in labour.

It is widely recognised that the more active a woman is during her pregnancy, the easier it will be for her to adapt to the changes to her body shape and increased weight as her pregnancy advances. Moderate exercise has been recognised as being beneficial to the healthy pregnant woman with an uncomplicated pregnancy, with no links to impaired foetal growth.

A pregnancy exercise programme helps women to be active, as far as is possible, during labour. Upright postures encourage utilisation of gravity, which may improve foetal descent in addition to improved alignment of the foetus for the passage through the pelvis. Also, there may be stronger and more efficient uterine contractions, reducing the risk of labour dystocia (slowing down or cessation of cervical dilatation). However, research also shows that women are less likely to assume positions that are unfamiliar to them to keep them upright/active. Squatting, kneeling or hands and knees positions may need some antenatal exploration. This is where pregnancy exercise classes also help to familiarise women with these positions.

In my experience, labouring women who have attended pregnancy exercise classes tend to be physically stronger, and more effective at breathing, relaxation and pushing techniques. These women tend to be more knowledgeable about how their bodies work and more in tune with the labouring process. This reduces tension, fear and anxiety – which makes your body work more effectively.

Emma Thorpe, Bsc (Hons) Midwifery
RGN, Ealing Hospital
www.emmasmidwiferyservices.co.uk

My final message to you before you deliver your precious child, no matter what your pregnancy has been like, no matter what mixed emotions you may be feeling, can only be this:
Go with the flow
Don't rule anything out

Give yourself permission to change your mind
Be yourself, don't be afraid to make a noise
If you need help, take it, don't be a martyr!
And most of all, accept the many moments labour presents you with: this is progress to the greatest achievement of your life.
Go on girl, you can do this! And we are all behind you!

Marie Behenna

PS Why not tell me all about your delivery via Twitter? Follow Fitmama1 and help other women to feel brave too!

Repair, eat and be happy!

CHAPTER 16

Skinny jeans? Forget it! First things first

So you've survived the birth of your baby. But you may not yet be past the train-smash that is the first six weeks of motherhood. There may be days when you don't even manage to get dressed before 2 pm, let alone find time to exercise and get back into shape.

We are under huge pressure via the media to have our babies and look like celebrities, wearing skinny jeans and looking glamorous, pushing our buggies as though we have not a care in the world.

Well, mums, I'm here to tell you that life is simply not like that! You are not superwoman, as much as you make a great impersonation of her. You are an exhausted, proud, stunned and normal mother, who has some priorities to get in check:

- Your baby needs you more than your skinny jeans do.
- Your body has been through an amazing journey, and needs time to recover.
- You do not have to be dressed before lunch if your day is not working out like that!
- You need to nourish yourself well so that you can care for your baby. Follow the same healthy eating plan as you did during pregnancy and you will be sure of good nourishment. This will enable you to cope with the exhaustion and stress of motherhood.
- You do not have to breastfeed. I am a great promoter of 'happy mummy = happy baby'. If breastfeeding has not happened for you and your baby, it is not the end of the

world. I was bottle-fed, my sister was breastfed, and we are both normal healthy adults who have gone on to have our own babies. Mine breastfed, and hers bottle-fed. Guess what? They're all normal, happy and as intelligent as one another!

- Your other half may not understand what you are going through at home, especially as their 'normal' life resumes when their paternity leave ends. Speak up and make sure they understand how you feel, without sounding like a crazy banshee. That is usually a sign of exhaustion anyway, so try to be calm when you ask for help.

- You do not have to attend every social mother and baby club going. Pick a couple that you would like to look forward to each week, and keep some days for you and your baby to just have quietly at home. Too many clubs and outings make for exhausted mums and cranky babies.

- If family and friends want to descend on you for visits, ask them to help with a couple of chores, like folding laundry while you natter, or get them to make the coffee while you feed your baby. Don't be a slave to visitors.

THE FITMAMA™ EARLY PELVIC FLOOR EXERCISES

The most important exercises in early postnatal recovery are for your pelvic floor group. It is important to repair these muscles before attempting more intense exercise. If you avoid doing this, you will set yourself up for further damage to the pelvic floor group. This kind of damage will potentially lead to prolapse of the pelvic organs, which can mean incontinence of varying degrees.

Pelvic floor exercises can be done as soon as you feel ready after your baby is born. Some passionate pelvic floor enthusiasts have been known to begin these on the day of delivery. You can still do them even if you are a caesarean mum.

In the first six weeks, I recommend that the only unsupervised exercise you take part in is:

a. functional walking with your baby in the buggy or sling;
b. pelvic floor and abdominal core repair.

The following pelvic floor exercises are suitable for the first six weeks of your baby's life outside your womb. Combine them with a gentle walking plan with your buggy to help get your natural endorphins flowing to beat the baby blues. Endorphins are produced by cells in your body when you exercise. They are the body's natural pain relievers and bring about a feeling of happiness and wellbeing.

Please only do these exercises if you are feeling well, and you are not suffering any postnatal complications. If you are in any doubt, it is always advisable to ask your health visitor or midwife if you are able to participate in these exercises.

THE PELVIC TILT

If you feel up to it, the pelvic tilt can be done in your hospital bed on the day of your delivery. If the thought has not even crossed your mind, please try to do this exercise within the first week of delivery.

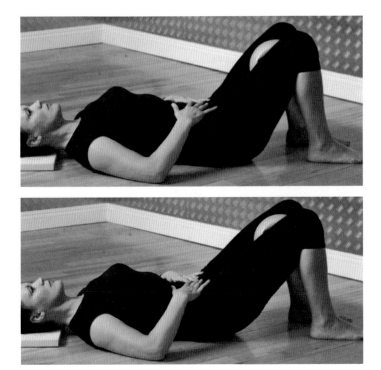

The pelvic tilt

Perform the exercise

Lie in a natural position on your back, keeping your back in comfortable alignment, your head resting on a cushion or pillow.

Place your hands over your lower abdomen to help you connect your mind to the pelvic floor.

Inhale to prepare.

Exhale to tidy up the bladder and back passage, and tilt the tailbone or bottom away from the floor.

Keep your back on the floor.

Repetition

As a guide, repeat this exercise 10 times, 3 times per day.

Top tip: You can place a soft ball or cushion between your thighs to help activate the pelvic floor muscles naturally, as, in the early days, you may find it difficult to feel the squeeze sensation. You can do this in bed too!

THE PELVIC LEG EXTENSION

Lie in a natural, comfortable position on your back, your head resting on a cushion or pillow. Start with knees together, feet flat on the floor and not placed wider than your pelvis.

Inhale to prepare.

Exhale to tidy up the bladder and back passage as you extend your leg slowly away from the body.

Extend your leg fully.

Inhale.

Exhale to return leg to start position.

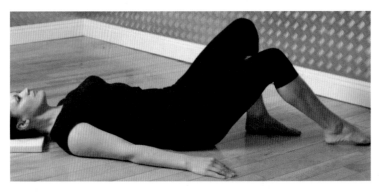

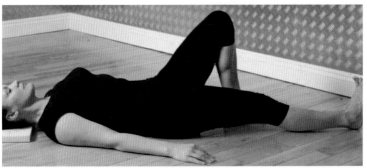

The pelvic leg extension

Repetition

As a guide, repeat this exercise 5–10 times per leg, 3 times a day.

Top tip: This is another exercise which can be done in bed. Try to ensure that the leg you are not sliding out stays still and does not waver from side to side.

You should be prepared to do pelvic floor exercises for the rest of your life to continue enjoying safe posture and good pelvic health, particularly if you are planning more children.

When you have made some progress towards repairing your pelvic floor and are feeling stronger and better able to cope after 6 weeks (12 if you had a caesarean section or other traumatic birth experience), you will be ready to try some more challenging postnatal exercise with a fully qualified postnatal exercise specialist. In the UK you can search for someone suitable in your area by contacting the Guild of Pregnancy and Postnatal Exercise Instructors. Not only will this help you progress safely, but you are likely to make some new friends who are going through the same sleepless nights as you are!

POSTNATAL WEIGHT AND DIET

When it comes to losing your pregnancy weight, hopefully you will not have gained too much if you have followed our healthy eating guidelines. However, if you have put on extra weight and are worried about losing it, I advise you not to follow extreme diets in the first year of your motherhood. Your body will need careful nourishment and care to help you cope. By the same token, you must try not to live on biscuits and easy-to-eat muffins (or whatever your guilty pleasure is). As an exhausted busy mum, you may find that easier said than done.

Here are a few simple solutions:

- Keep carrot sticks and hummous in the fridge for easy snacking.
- Fruit and nuts are the answer when cakes are staring at you from the cupboard.
- When cooking meals, make a little extra to keep in the fridge or freezer as leftovers to quickly heat up.
- Chocolate and sugar cravings are directly associated with lack of sleep, so try to take a good all-round supplement which includes magnesium. This will help you cope with exhaustion and combat sweet cravings.

- Vitamin C may help you to keep bugs at bay while your immunity is rebuilt following the challenge of labour.
- Omega oils may help your joints recover from the strains of pregnancy weight, and are good for your overloaded brain cells too!
- Protein is good for tissue repair, so eat plenty of lean meat, fish and beans.

Most of all, enjoy your baby, worship your amazing body (whatever shape it is in right now), and promise yourself to ask for help if you need it. Keep moving, keep eating well, keep breathing, find time for relaxation with your baby, and be a true FitMama™!

CONFIDENCE AFFIRMATIONS FOR POSTNATAL MUMS

- I am a strong and capable woman.
- My body knows how to repair itself.
- My baby is thriving and feels my love.
- My natural maternal instincts guide me every day.
- I nourish my body with healthy food and water.
- I nourish my baby with milk and love.
- I am calm.
- My body can cope with these broken nights.
- I love my postnatal body.
- I accept the changes to my body.
- I embrace my stretch marks as the markers of my incredible journey into motherhood.
- I accept that my baby will sometimes cry without easy consolation.
- I accept that some days will not go to plan, and that is okay!
- I embrace the days I do not get out of my pyjamas until lunchtime because the day has not gone to plan.
- I love my partner.
- My partner loves me and my changed postnatal body.
- I embrace advice, and make my own choices.
- I trust my instincts to protect my baby.
- I am a mother, a lover, a friend, and I am still me.

CHAPTER 17

Barbara Bradbury's holistic recipes for pregnancy

Barbara Bradbury, my friend, fellow professional, naturopathic nutritional therapist, life and performance coach, has kindly shared her healing recipes for pregnancy with me so that I can give you some ideas about eating well for you and your baby during these wonderful months. You can follow more of Barbara's nutritional treats on her website www.shapingupforlife.co.uk

As much as it's easy to opt for naughty food because you feel you no longer need to suck in your tummy, please try these healthier options as they are not only delicious but also good for both of you.

I also encourage you to use those last dragging days of pregnancy to create some of these dishes, freeze them, and keep them for those early days of parenthood when both you and your partner may feel too overwhelmed to even think about cooking. Plus, it means that you can spend more time getting into a routine with your newborn, and still have time to eat nourishing healthy food. Nutrition is paramount to your recovery, so get ahead of the game, cook up these delights, and freeze them for an easy, healthy life!

BREAKFAST RECIPES

Vanilla yogurt muesli breakfast
Serves 1
Preparation: 5 minutes

Ingredients
4 oz organic sheep's yogurt (easier to digest) *or* organic yogurt
   substitute, if on a dairy-free diet
1 tsp wild organic or raw honey
A few drops of pure vanilla extract
2 tbsp organic oats or gluten free muesli or cereal
Banana, apple, pear, berries e.g. blueberries/raspberries, mango,
   kiwifruit
Optional: Nuts: almonds (soaked overnight and skins removed),
brazil nuts, hazelnuts (soaked overnight). Seeds: dark green
pumpkin seeds

Method
Mix the yoghurt and your choice of accompaniments in a bowl.
The organic oats will provide some slow-release glucose
carbohydrates.

Health information
Protein builds, repairs and maintains cells in your body. Protein manufactures haemoglobin, which is red blood cells that carry oxygen;
also manufactures antibodies to fight disease and illness.

(*Note:* If you have a dairy intolerance, soak almonds overnight, peel
off the skins and liquidise to make an almond milk which you can
use instead of dairy milk.)

Porridge with fruit

Serves 1
Preparation: 5 minutes
Cooking time: 10 minutes

Ingredients

10 fl oz organic milk substitute
3 oz organic porridge oats
1 tbsp raisins
1 organic apple (chopped)
Optional: 1 tsp cinnamon or mixed spice; other fruits of your choice such as pear or raspberries

Method

1. Place the porridge oats with the milk substitute into a saucepan. Bring to the boil, stirring frequently (you can add a little water if too thick), then reduce the heat to medium, add the raisins and simmer for a few minutes.
2. Wash the apple and chop up into pieces and add to the porridge. Add optional spices or other fruit of your choice; mix well.

Health information

Porridge oats are a good source of soluble fibre, which softens the stools in the bowels, helping to eliminate waste more efficiently. Soluble fibre slows down digestion and the sudden release of glucose into the bloodstream provides us with consistent levels of energy. Porridge oats are also good for weight balance as when the glucose is released, moderate levels of insulin are released. If you have a gluten intolerance, irritable bowel syndrome or other bowel problems use millet flakes instead (earthier taste, but if you add fruit and a little honey to sweeten you won't notice).

LUNCH RECIPES

Egg and potato salad
Serves 4
Preparation time: 15 minutes

Ingredients
2 lb cooked new potatoes or winter potatoes (with skins on)
1 small onion, finely shredded, *or* 4 large spring onions, shredded
6 hard-boiled free range organic eggs
6 tbsp tahini dressing
Optional: 2 tbsp fresh parsley, finely chopped, *or* 1 tsp mild paprika

Method
1. Chop the cooked potatoes into bite size pieces and mix with the shredded onions in a large bowl.
2. Chop up 4 of the eggs, reserving the other 2 for decoration, and add to the potatoes and onion.
3. Mix in the dressing, then decorate with the 2 leftover eggs by cutting into quarters and placing around the top of the potato salad.
4. Sprinkle over some finely chopped fresh parsley or the tsp of paprika, or both.
Serve with a freshly made green salad.

Health information
Eggs contain many nutrients, including vitamins A, D (helps calcium absorption), calcium, iron, choline, which are all important nutrients for a healthy pregnant mother. Tahini (sesame seed paste; try to purchase raw tahini) is rich in calcium and contains minerals such as magnesium, zinc and vitamin E. If you are on a dairy-free or fat-free diet I would suggest you take vitamin D3 supplements, but

please check with your doctor first. Also, check with your doctor that you are taking enough folic acid.

Carrot and cauliflower salad

Serves 2-4
Preparation time: 15 minutes
Cooking time: 3 minutes

Ingredients
8 oz organic carrots, grated
8 oz cauliflower florets
1 large onion, shredded
2 tbsp Italian dressing or dressing of your choice

Method
1. Steam or blanch the cauliflower florets and onion for a few minutes then put under cold running water.
2) Place the cauliflower in a salad bowl with the grated carrots and mix in the dressing.
Serve with lentils bolognese, meat or fish

Health information
Cauliflower contains indoles and isothiocyanates, which are plant chemicals that have disease-preventive properties. All vegetables and fruits contain different types of disease-preventing phytochemicals, which is why it's a good idea to eat a varied diet containing all the colours of the rainbow from vegetables, salad and fruit.

Broccoli, carrot, tomato and dill salad

Serves 2
Preparation time: 15 minutes
Cooking time: 3 minutes

Ingredients
6 oz broccoli florets
6 oz organic carrots, grated
3-4 organic tomatoes
1 small red onion, shredded

4 tbsp basic or garlic dressing
2 tbsp chopped dill
Optional: dark green pumpkin seeds or sunflower seeds

Method

1. Steam the broccoli for a few minutes, then put under cold running water and set aside.
2. Mix all of the ingredients together and gently toss until the salad is covered in the dressing.
3. Sprinkle the seeds, if you are using them, over the salad.

Serve with tabbouleh, meat, fish, egg omelette, egg and potato salad or vegan food.

Health information

Steaming broccoli is the best way to cook it. Broccoli is rich in beta carotene (good for eyesight) and phytonutrients which help the body's detoxification system. Tomatoes are rich in calcium, potassium, phosphorous and beta carotene, and they contain a phytochemical called lycopene, an antioxidant which could help fight cancer. The seeds contain essential fatty acids (EFAs) and extra minerals and vitamin E.

Lentil and vegetable soup

Serves 2
Preparation time: 10-15 minutes
Cooking time: 20 minutes

Ingredients

4 oz orange or green lentils
2 onions, chopped
4 large carrots, chopped
4 sticks celery, chopped
2 cloves of garlic, crushed
2 pints of water, or enough water to cover the ingredients
Optional: a pinch of pink Himalayan crystal salt; 1 tsp onion seeds and ½ tsp celery seeds; 1-2 tsp dried herbs or 1-2 tbsp fresh herbs; 1 tbsp lemon dressing

Method

1. If you are using green lentils you will need to cook them for 15 minutes first; if using red lentils, they can cook with the vegetables. (If you suffer flatulence problems with lentils you can sprout them before you cook them; this will take a couple of days.)

2. Put all the ingredients (except the herbs and lemon dressing) and the water into a large saucepan, bring to the boil and simmer for 15 minutes or until the vegetables are soft and tender.

3. Put the soup ingredients into a blender with the herbs (if using) and/or lemon dressing and blend until smooth. If using fresh herbs you may wish to sprinkle some on top of your soup for decoration.

Serve with spelt or rye bread. If you are on a gluten-free diet you can add some cooked rice or cooked quinoa (you cook it like couscous).

Health information

Pulses (which include lentils) are a cheap source of protein and also contain fibre and iron. Use a little pink Himalayan crystal salt instead of white table salt as this salt contains 84 minerals and trace elements which help the body to function well and is much healthier than white salt. It is said this salt also contains ancient energy, so a little now and again is good for you.

MAIN MEALS

Chicken tagine

Serves 4

Preparation time: about 30 minutes
Cooking time: it takes about 2 hours to cook the chicken and 45 minutes to cook the tagine.

Ingredients
1 medium-size free range or organic chicken
2 oz unsalted butter
3 onions
3 large cloves of garlic, crushed
1 organic vegetable stock cube
1 pint of water
1 large pinch saffron
1-inch piece of root ginger, finely chopped
1 tbsp paprika
½ tsp cinnamon
4 oz organic apricots, washed and cut in half or kept whole
12 oz broad beans *or* chopped green beans
6 turns of freshly-milled black pepper
2 tbsp fresh coriander, finely chopped
2 tbsp fresh parsley, finely chopped

Method
1. Cook the chicken, following the cooking instructions on the packaging. This should take around 2 hours if using a 3-lb chicken.
2. Once cooked, pull away all the cooked chicken from the bone, cover and set aside.
3. Peel and chop one of the onions into rings and finely chop the other two. Put the onions into a large saucepan with the butter

and fry on a moderate heat for 5 minutes, then add the garlic and cook for a further 3 minutes.

4. Next add the pint of water, the stock cube, chicken, saffron, root ginger, paprika, and cinnamon. Stir, bring to the boil then simmer for 20 minutes.

5. Add the apricots, broad beans or green beans and black pepper and simmer for another 15 minutes.

6. Mix in the herbs and upon serving sprinkle some parsley on top for decoration.

Serve with cooked rice, gluten-free pasta, potato and quinoa (if food combining) and salad or vegetables or both. This dish has a subtle flavour so children should like it – just make sure you've removed all the chicken bones.

Health information

Dried apricots promote good heart and eye health and contain zeaxanthin, a phytochemical which helps protect eyes from age-related macular disease. They also contain the minerals potassium, iron, zinc, calcium, copper and manganese. Potassium and magnesium are good for maintaining a healthy heart.

(*Note:* If you have children who do not like apricots, you can cut the apricots into smaller pieces and add them at the beginning of cooking time; they will then melt a bit and the children will probably not notice them.)

Lamb shepherd's pie

Serves 4
Preparation time: 30 minutes
Cooking time: 40-45 minutes

Ingredients
Topping
2 lb potatoes
8 oz soft carrots *or* squash *or* parsnips *or* ½ cooked potatoes and ½ sweet potatoes
2 oz organic unsalted butter

Filling
1 lb lean minced lamb
1 tbsp extra virgin olive oil
1 large onion, chopped
2 cooked carrots, chopped
6 oz garden peas
4 oz mushrooms (optional)
3 cloves of crushed garlic
2 tsp mixed herbs
1 tin organic chopped tomatoes
½ jar organic tomato purée

Method
1. Pre-heat oven to gas mark 5, 375°F, 190°C.
2. *Filling*: Cook the onion in a frying pan with the olive oil for 4 minutes then add the lamb and cook for a further 6 minutes, stirring the mixture frequently. Add the garlic and cook for another couple of minutes.
3. Add the herbs, carrots, tinned chopped tomatoes, garden peas and simmer for another 10 minutes. Add the tomato purée and cook for a further couple of minutes.
4. *Topping*: Cook the potatoes in about 1½ pints of water until tender. You could cook the carrots with the potatoes or simply steam the carrots. When they are both soft, purée the carrots with the butter and a little hot water in a liquidiser. If your mixture is too thick, add some more hot water.
5. Drain away the water from the potatoes and mash in the carrot purée. Set aside.
6. Spread the lamb mixture over the base of a large ovenproof casserole dish then gently spread the potato mash over the top. Fluff up the surface with a fork and put some tiny knobs of butter over the surface of the pie. Bake in the oven for 30 minutes until golden brown on top.
Serve with salad or vegetables or both.

Health information
Red meat is the richest source of absorbable iron. Iron is essential for cell respiration and metabolism, energy metabolism, DNA synthesis, neurological development, red blood cell formation, growth and healing, benefitting mother and baby.

Fish with jacket potatoes

Serves 2
Preparation time: 10 minutes
Cooking time: 30 minutes

Ingredients
2 sea bream, redfish or sea bass, cleaned and trimmed
2 large potatoes, skin on
A little unsalted butter

Method
1. Pre-heat oven to gas mark 6, 400°F, 200°C.
2. Slice the potatoes in half and brush a little of the butter over each half. Lightly butter a roasting tin and place the potatoes in it. Put into the oven and cook for about 10 minutes.
3. Add the fish and cook for another 30 minutes or until cooked through. If cooking redfish instead of sea bream you can slice some lemon and squeeze over the fish.

Serve with salad or vegetables or both.

Health information
Fish is an excellent source of omega-3 fatty acids, which are excellent for a healthy brain and nervous system. O3 is also good for eyesight, and for making hormones which control your bodily functions. Eating fish during pregnancy may reduce the risk of a premature baby; however, choose the low mercury options. The general rule of thumb during pregnancy is a couple of portions of fish a week.

HEALTHY SWEET TREATS

Apple and cinnamon muesli biscuits
Preparation time 15-20 minutes
Cooking time: 15-20 minutes
Makes: about 24 biscuits

Ingredients
2 oz unsalted butter
1 tbsp organic honey or rice syrup or maple syrup
4 oz molasses sugar
4 oz organic apricots or dates, chopped
1 egg
5 oz organic buckwheat flakes
5 oz organic millet flakes or 10 oz organic oats
8 oz gluten-free flour or organic spelt flour
4 oz organic almonds or cashew nuts, chopped
3 organic apples, grated
4 tsp cinnamon

Method
1. Pre-heat oven to gas mark 6, 400°F, 200°C.
2. Blend together in a food processor the butter, honey, molasses, apricots and egg.
3. Put the flakes, gluten-free flour, almonds, grated apples and cinnamon into a bowl and mix in the blended butter, honey etc. until the mixture has amalgamated.
4. Lightly butter a non-stick baking tray and press the mixture into the tray until about 1 cm thick. You can use a floured rolling pin to flatten the mixture.
5. Bake in the oven for 15-20 minutes or until cooked through.

Health information

If you think you have a gluten intolerance, or your child has, it is worth replacing wheat flour with gluten-free flour. Organic spelt flour is worth trying as it can be tolerated and will have more fibre, B vitamins and minerals. The symptoms of gluten intolerance are irritable bowel syndrome, erratic behaviour or mood swings, inability to relax.

Date or apricot and toasted almond snack bars

Preparation time: 15 minutes
Cooking time: 5 minutes
Refrigeration time: 2 hours
Makes: 10-12 snack bars

Ingredients

1 cup of dates or organic apricots
½ mug of apple juice
3 oz ground flaxseed
3 oz very lightly toasted almonds

Method

1. Cook the dates or apricots in the apple juice for 5 minutes, until a smooth mixture is formed.
2. Chop the lightly toasted almonds in a food processor and set aside in a dish.
3. Put the ground flaxseed (grind in a coffee or nut grinder) and date or apricot mixture into the food processor and blend until a dough is formed. Then add the almonds and blend again until all the ingredients are mixed.
4. Oil a flat dish and press the mixture down firmly; it should be about ¼ inch deep.
5. Refrigerate for 2 hours then cut into little rectangles.
Note: These are very healthy for children as well.

Health information

Flaxseed contains lignans which are great for bowel health and are known to help prevent bowel cancer. It's an excellent idea to ingest flaxseed (golden linseed) during pregnancy as this will help the passing of stools (particularly after childbirth, when you're still tender down below). It is better to ingest flaxseeds ground, either in food as in these snack bars or as a tea. See below for my healing flaxseed/linseed tea.

Almonds contain vitamin E, magnesium, manganese, phosphorus, vitamin B2, copper, potassium and calcium.

Healing flaxseed/linseed tea
Preparation time: 5 minutes

Ingredients
1 tbsp flaxseed/golden linseed
Water

Method
1. Boil a kettle of water.
2. Grind the flaxseed/linseed in a coffee or nut grinder and put into a mug. Pour on enough cold water to make a loose paste.
3. When the kettle has boiled pour in the hot water, stir and drink within 10 minutes.

Health information
See the health information for the snack bars above for the properties of flaxseed/linseed. The great aspect of this drink is that when you have just given birth and you feel very sore down below you will feel great comfort knowing it's easier to pass stools.

ACKNOWLEDGEMENTS

There are a number of people I would like to thank and acknowledge.

- Natalie Melton, without whom none of this would have been so easy. Natalie, thank you for your faith in the FitMama™ mission, and for the work you have done with us to raise the profile of FitMama™, all of which led to this publication.
- Mr Ernest Hecht of Souvenir Press, an inspirational man who has opened the door to me and given me a platform from which to spout forth my opinions!
- Lola Turvey, my right-hand lady, for her patience and humour during the long and hot photo shoot for the photographs in this book, and her ongoing commitment to FitMama™ participants everywhere.
- Gemma Dedman, for her photographs of Lola Turvey and her patience with my pernickety direction: www.gemmadedman.co.uk
- Carli Adby for the photographs of the FitMama™ classes: www.adbycreative.co.uk
- Georgina Wilson and Barbara Bradbury for their nutritional contributions.
- Thanks to Emma Thorpe for her advice about and support of the content of this book. www.emmasmidwiferyservices.co.uk
- Wendy Daly, Julie Honour, Karen Middleton and Lola Turvey for their contributions and personal photographs.
- Katerina Kolenova, the model on the cover.
- FitMama™ participants who contributed via our Facebook pages to share their experiences with you.
- Canadian Society for Exercise Physiology: www.csep.ca

- Royal College of Obstetricians and Gynaecologists: www.rcog.org.uk
- National Centre for Eating Disorders: www.eating-disorders.org.uk
- www.hypermobility.org/pregnancy.php
- www.nhs.uk/Conditions/Joint-hypermobility
- www.nhs.uk/conditions/Marfan-syndrome
- www.ehlers-danlos.org
- www.marfan.org/marfan
- Thanks to my lovely family for their ongoing support and help with my children during the busiest time of my life.

Everyone needs a soul mate . . . mine offered me encouragement and faith in my ability to complete this project.
My paperweight.

The Fitmama™ Instructor Training Programme

Certified fitness professionals have the opportunity to become fully qualified Fitmama™ Trainers. Learn how to teach The Fitmama™ Method to women in your community through this REPs recognised qualification.

Enquiries accepted via the official Fitmama™ website: www.fitmama.org

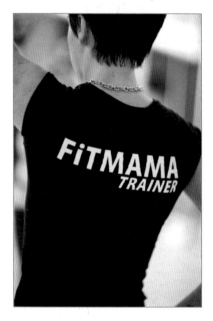

Courses are available to help you achieve the relevant qualifications required to enrol on the Fitmama™ Instructor Training Programme. In association with Careers in Fitness Ltd.

CONTACT:
Twitter: @fitmama1
Facebook: The Fitmama Method
Web: www.thefitmamamethod.com